Alzheimer's chronicles

Understanding , batting and conquering Alzheimer's within

BY

Dr. Austin lerry

Copyright

TABLE OF CONTENT

Introduction

Alzheimer's disease, a name that strikes fear and uncertainty into the hearts of millions, stands as one of the most formidable challenges facing modern healthcare. It is a relentless and enigmatic foe, gradually eroding the essence of the human self – memory, cognition, and identity. In this exploration of Alzheimer's, we embark on a journey into the depths of a disease that knows no boundaries, affecting individuals regardless of age, gender, or background. It is a journey that begins with understanding not only the disease itself but also the profound impact it has on individuals, families, and society as a whole.

At its core, Alzheimer's is a neurological disorder, a thief that steals not only memories but also the essence of who we are. To unravel its intricacies, we must first peer into the remarkable complexity of the human brain, an organ of unfathomable beauty and intricacy. This is the foundation upon which our understanding of Alzheimer's disease is built.

The brain, often likened to the universe within, is the command center of human existence. It orchestrates every thought, every emotion, every movement. In **Chapter 2: Brain Health and Aging**, we embark on a voyage into the inner workings of this magnificent organ. We explore the delicate balance that underlies our cognitive abilities and how, with the passage of time, the brain undergoes changes that are a natural part of aging. Yet, Alzheimer's is no natural part of this process. It is a disrupter of this balance, a rogue force that alters the landscape of our neurological terrain.

As we venture further into the chapters that follow, we will unravel the mysteries of Alzheimer's disease, from its causes and risk factors to the heart-wrenching journey of caregiving. We will delve into the scientific quest for a cure and the promising developments on the horizon. Moreover, we will seek to understand not only the disease's clinical aspects but also the human stories that illuminate its impact.

This book is more than an exploration of a medical condition; it is a testament to the resilience of the human spirit, the unwavering dedication of caregivers, and the unyielding pursuit of knowledge and hope in the face of adversity. It is a guide, a source of solace, and a beacon of understanding for those touched by Alzheimer's, directly or indirectly. So, let us embark on this voyage together, as we endeavor to shed light on the shadows cast by Alzheimer's disease, and find the strength to face the challenges it presents with compassion, knowledge, and empathy.

Chapter 1

What is Alzheimer's?

Alzheimer's disease is a devastating and progressive neurodegenerative disorder that primarily affects the brain, causing a decline in cognitive function and memory. Named after Dr. Alois Alzheimer, who first identified it in 1906, this condition is characterized by the accumulation of abnormal protein deposits in the brain, specifically beta-amyloid plaques and tau tangles. These inputs disrupt communication between brain cells, that leads to their breakdown and eventual death.

The hallmark symptoms of Alzheimer's include memory loss, confusion, disorientation, and difficulty in problem-solving and language comprehension. As the disease advances, individuals may experience personality changes, mood swings, and impaired motor function. Alzheimer's is typically diagnosed in older adults, although early-onset cases can affect individuals in their 40s and 50s.

While the exact cause of Alzheimer's remains unclear, genetics, age, and environmental factors are believed to contribute to its development. Currently, there is no cure for Alzheimer's disease, and available treatments aim to alleviate symptoms and slow down its progression. Research into potential therapies and interventions continues, with the hope of one day finding a cure or more effective treatments to address this global health challenge. Alzheimer's not only impacts the individuals suffering from it but also places a significant emotional and caregiving burden on their families and caregivers. As the aging population grows, understanding and addressing Alzheimer's remains a critical area of research and healthcare focus.

Historical Perspective

The historical perspective of Alzheimer's disease traces back over a century and reflects the evolving understanding of this complex neurological disorder.

1. Discovery by Alois Alzheimer (1906):
Alzheimer's disease was first identified by the German neurologist Dr. Alois Alzheimer in 1906. He documented the case of Auguste Deter, a woman who exhibited severe memory loss, disorientation, and unusual behavioral changes. Upon her death, Dr. Alzheimer conducted a post-mortem examination of her brain and discovered abnormal protein deposits, now known as beta-amyloid plaques and tau tangles. This groundbreaking discovery laid the foundation for future research into the disease.

2. Early Theories and Nomenclature:
In the early 20th century, Alzheimer's disease was often referred to as "presenile dementia" due to its occurrence in younger individuals. The term "Alzheimer's disease" became widely accepted in the medical community, and it was recognized as a distinct form of dementia.

3. Advancements in Research (20th Century):
Throughout the 20th century, research into Alzheimer's disease expanded. Researchers developed a better understanding of its

clinical presentation and neuropathological characteristics. The development of neuroimaging techniques allowed for in vivo observation of brain changes in affected individuals.

4. Cholinergic Hypothesis and Medications:
In the 1970s, the cholinergic hypothesis proposed that a deficiency in the neurotransmitter acetylcholine played a significant role in Alzheimer's disease. This led to the development of cholinesterase inhibitors, such as donepezil, which are still used today to treat cognitive symptoms.

5. Genetic Discoveries (1980s-1990s):
The identification of genetic mutations associated with familial forms of Alzheimer's disease, such as mutations in the APP, PSEN1, and PSEN2 genes, provided crucial insights into the disease's genetic basis. These discoveries paved the way for genetic testing and a better understanding of sporadic cases.

6. Global Impact and Advocacy:
As the prevalence of Alzheimer's disease increased with aging populations worldwide, it gained recognition as a significant public health issue. Advocacy groups and organizations like the Alzheimer's Association emerged to raise awareness, support research, and provide resources for patients and caregivers.

7. Ongoing Research and Therapeutic Developments:
In recent decades, research efforts have intensified, focusing on unraveling the molecular mechanisms underlying Alzheimer's disease. While there is still no cure, promising advancements in drug development, including anti-amyloid and anti-tau therapies, offer hope for more effective treatments and potential disease-modifying interventions.

The historical perspective of Alzheimer's disease reflects a journey from its initial discovery by Alois Alzheimer to ongoing efforts to understand, diagnose, and ultimately find a cure for this challenging condition. As our knowledge continues to expand, the goal remains to improve the quality of life for individuals affected by Alzheimer's and their families.

Science of Alzheimer's

The science of Alzheimer's disease is a complex and multifaceted field of research aimed at understanding the underlying causes, mechanisms, and potential treatments for this debilitating neurodegenerative condition. Here, we delve into the key aspects of the science of Alzheimer's:

1. Pathological Hallmarks:
Alzheimer's disease is characterized by two primary pathological hallmarks - beta-amyloid plaques and tau tangles. Beta-amyloid plaques are formed from the accumulation of beta-amyloid protein fragments between nerve cells, while tau tangles are twisted tangles of tau protein within nerve cells. These abnormal protein deposits disrupt neuronal function and lead to cell death.

2. Neuroinflammation:
Chronic neuroinflammation is a prominent feature of Alzheimer's. Microglia, the brain's immune cells, become activated and release

inflammatory molecules in response to the presence of beta-amyloid plaques and other pathological changes. This inflammatory response can further damage neurons and exacerbate cognitive decline.

3. Genetics:

While the majority of Alzheimer's cases are sporadic, certain genetic mutations are associated with a higher risk of developing the disease. Mutations in genes such as APP, PSEN1, and PSEN2 are linked to early-onset familial Alzheimer's, providing insights into the role of these genes in beta-amyloid production and processing.

4. Amyloid Hypothesis:

The amyloid hypothesis posits that the accumulation of beta-amyloid plaques is a primary trigger for Alzheimer's disease. Researchers have developed various therapeutic strategies targeting beta-amyloid, including monoclonal antibodies designed to remove these plaques.

5. Tau Hypothesis:

The tau hypothesis suggests that the abnormal aggregation of tau protein is another critical factor in Alzheimer's progression. Aberrant tau tangles disrupt the microtubules responsible for maintaining the structural integrity of neurons, leading to cell dysfunction and death. Therapies targeting tau are also under investigation.

6. Early Detection:

Efforts to detect Alzheimer's disease in its early stages have intensified. Biomarkers, including cerebrospinal fluid proteins and neuroimaging techniques like PET scans, are being explored to identify the disease before significant cognitive impairment occurs.

7. Therapeutic Developments:
While there is currently no cure for Alzheimer's, ongoing research has led to the development of symptomatic treatments like cholinesterase inhibitors and NMDA receptor antagonists. Additionally, numerous clinical trials are testing potential disease-modifying therapies aimed at altering the course of the disease by targeting beta-amyloid, tau, or other mechanisms.

8. Holistic Approaches:
Researchers are increasingly recognizing the importance of a holistic approach to Alzheimer's management. Lifestyle factors such as diet, exercise, cognitive stimulation, and social engagement may help mitigate the risk of developing the disease or slow its progression.

The science of Alzheimer's disease is a dynamic field that continues to evolve as researchers strive to unlock the mysteries of this devastating condition. While many questions remain, advances in our understanding of the disease's biology hold promise for the development of more effective treatments and, ultimately, a cure.

Chapter 2:

Brain Health and Aging

Brain health and aging are closely intertwined with Alzheimer's disease, a condition that primarily affects older individuals. Understanding the relationship between brain aging and Alzheimer's is essential for both prevention and treatment strategies.

1. Normal Brain Aging:
As people age, their brains naturally undergo changes. These changes include a slight decrease in brain volume and a decline in processing speed and working memory. These age-related changes are considered normal and typically do not severely impair daily functioning.

2. Alzheimer's and Abnormal Brain Aging:
Alzheimer's disease represents an extreme form of abnormal brain aging. In Alzheimer's, there is a significant accumulation of beta-amyloid plaques and tau tangles, which disrupt the normal functioning of neurons. This abnormal aging process leads to severe cognitive impairment, including memory loss, confusion, and difficulty with daily tasks.

3. Risk Factors:
Several risk factors contribute to the relationship between aging and Alzheimer's disease. Advanced age itself is the most significant risk factor, with the incidence of Alzheimer's increasing exponentially after the age of 65. Genetics, family history, and certain lifestyle factors, such as poor diet, lack of exercise, and limited cognitive engagement, also influence the risk of developing the disease.

4. Protective Factors:
Conversely, there are protective factors that can promote brain health and potentially delay the onset of Alzheimer's. Regular physical activity, a balanced diet rich in antioxidants and omega-3 fatty acids, social engagement, and mentally stimulating activities like puzzles and learning new skills may help preserve cognitive function as individuals age.

5. Neuroplasticity:
The brain retains a degree of plasticity, or the ability to reorganize and form new neural connections throughout life. Engaging in activities that challenge the brain, such as learning a new language or musical instrument, can promote cognitive reserve, which may delay the manifestation of Alzheimer's symptoms.

6. Early Detection and Intervention:
Early detection of Alzheimer's is crucial for effective intervention. Biomarkers, neuroimaging, and cognitive assessments are tools that can help identify the disease in its early stages, allowing for early intervention and better outcomes.

7. Lifestyle Choices:
Promoting brain health through lifestyle choices is gaining prominence in Alzheimer's prevention. Adopting a Mediterranean-

style diet, maintaining cardiovascular health, managing chronic conditions like diabetes and hypertension, and staying mentally and socially active are all factors that can support healthy brain aging and reduce the risk of Alzheimer's.

In summary, while aging is a natural process that affects the brain, Alzheimer's represents a severe and abnormal form of brain aging. Understanding the risk factors and protective factors associated with both aging and Alzheimer's is critical for promoting brain health and developing strategies to prevent or manage this devastating disease as the global population continues to age.

How the Brain Works

Alzheimer's disease profoundly impacts how the brain functions. To understand this, it's essential to explore how the brain works in the context of Alzheimer's:

1. Neuron Communication:
The brain relies on the intricate communication between billions of neurons (nerve cells). Neurons transmit electrical and chemical signals through synapses, the tiny gaps between them. These signals enable thoughts, emotions, and motor functions.

2. Beta-Amyloid Accumulation:
In Alzheimer's, beta-amyloid protein fragments accumulate outside neurons and form plaques. These plaques disrupt synaptic function, interfering with the transmission of signals between neurons. As a result, cognitive processes like memory and learning become impaired.

3. Tau Protein Abnormalities:
Tau proteins stabilize the internal structure of neurons by supporting microtubules. In Alzheimer's, tau proteins become abnormally phosphorylated and aggregate into neurofibrillary tangles within neurons. This disrupts the structural integrity of neurons, leading to their dysfunction and eventual death.

4. Neuroinflammation:
Chronic neuroinflammation is another aspect of how the brain works in Alzheimer's. Microglia, the brain's immune cells, become overactive and release inflammatory molecules in response to beta-amyloid plaques and tau tangles. This inflammation can cause further damage to neurons.

5. Cell Death and Brain Atrophy:
Over time, the accumulation of beta-amyloid plaques, tau tangles, and neuroinflammation results in neuronal death and brain atrophy, particularly in regions responsible for memory and cognition. This leads to the progressive cognitive decline seen in Alzheimer's patients.

6. Impaired Neurotransmission:
Neurotransmitters, chemical messengers, play a vital role in brain function. In Alzheimer's, the loss of synapses, along with the death of neurons, disrupts the balance of neurotransmitters like acetylcholine. This imbalance contributes to memory and cognitive deficits.

7. Disrupted Neural Networks:
The brain relies on complex neural networks for various functions. In Alzheimer's, these networks become disrupted due to the damage caused by beta-amyloid plaques, tau tangles, and cell

death. As a result, the brain struggles to process information, leading to cognitive impairment.

8. Cognitive and Behavioral Symptoms:
The culmination of these brain abnormalities manifests as Alzheimer's symptoms, including memory loss, confusion, personality changes, mood swings, and eventually, the inability to perform daily tasks independently.

Understanding how the brain works in Alzheimer's is essential for developing treatments that target the disease's underlying mechanisms. Current research aims to find ways to remove or reduce beta-amyloid and tau abnormalities, modulate neuroinflammation, and promote synaptic health. While there is no cure for Alzheimer's yet, advancements in our understanding of the disease offer hope for more effective treatments in the future.

Normal Aging vs. Alzheimer's

Normal aging and Alzheimer's disease are two distinct processes that affect cognitive function and overall well-being in different ways. Understanding the differences between them is crucial for early detection and appropriate care. Here's a comparison of normal aging and Alzheimer's:

1. Memory Changes:
Normal Aging: It's common for older adults to experience mild memory changes, such as occasionally forgetting names or

details. These memory lapses do not significantly impact daily life and are often attributed to age-related changes in brain function.

Alzheimer's: In Alzheimer's, memory loss is more severe and progressive. Individuals may forget essential information, such as names of family members or recent events, significantly affecting their ability to function independently.

2. Cognitive Function:

Normal Aging: Cognitive abilities, such as reasoning and problem-solving, may decline slightly with age but generally remain within a normal range. Older adults are able to make these changes.

Alzheimer's: Cognitive decline in Alzheimer's is more pronounced and relentless. Individuals may struggle with tasks they once performed easily, have difficulty with complex reasoning, and experience significant impairment in their daily lives.

3. Language Skills:

Normal Aging: Older adults may take slightly longer to recall words or articulate thoughts, but their language abilities remain intact.

Alzheimer's: In Alzheimer's, language difficulties are more noticeable, with individuals struggling to find words, repeating themselves, or losing the ability to follow or initiate conversations.

4. Spatial Awareness and Navigation:

Normal Aging: Mild declines in spatial awareness and navigation abilities can occur with age, but they usually do not result in significant problems.

Alzheimer's: Alzheimer's can lead to severe spatial disorientation, making it challenging for individuals to recognize familiar places and perform tasks like driving.

5. Independence:

Normal Aging: Older adults can generally maintain their independence and continue with their daily activities and responsibilities.

Alzheimer's: Alzheimer's progressively robs individuals of their independence as they struggle with basic tasks like dressing, eating, and bathing, eventually requiring full-time care.

6. Behavioral and Mood Changes:

Normal Aging: Mood changes in older adults are typically associated with life events or health issues but do not result in drastic personality changes.

Alzheimer's: Alzheimer's can cause significant mood swings, agitation, and personality changes, often leading to emotional distress for both the affected individual and their caregivers.

It's important to note that not all memory and cognitive changes in older adults indicate Alzheimer's disease. Many factors, including stress, depression, and medication side effects, can affect cognitive function. However, persistent and severe cognitive decline should be evaluated by a healthcare professional to rule out conditions like Alzheimer's disease. Early diagnosis and appropriate care can help manage the symptoms and improve the quality of life for individuals with Alzheimer's and their families.

Chapter 3

Causes and Risk Factor

Alzheimer's disease is a complex condition with multiple contributing factors. While the exact cause remains unclear, researchers have identified several causes and risk factors associated with the development of Alzheimer's:

1. Age:
Age is the most profound risk factor for Alzheimer's disease. The tendency of getting the condition increases significantly with an increase in age. While Alzheimer's can affect individuals in their 40s and 50s (early-onset Alzheimer's), it is primarily a disease of old age.

2. Genetics:
Genetic factors play a role in Alzheimer's disease. Mutations in specific genes, such as APP, PSEN1, and PSEN2, are linked to early-onset familial Alzheimer's. Additionally, the presence of the APOE ε4 allele is associated with an increased risk of developing the more common late-onset form of Alzheimer's.

3. Family History:
A family history of Alzheimer's disease raises the risk for developing the condition. Individuals with first-degree relatives (parents, siblings) who have had Alzheimer's are at a higher risk.

4. Beta-Amyloid Accumulation:
The accumulation of beta-amyloid plaques in the brain is a hallmark of Alzheimer's. Abnormal processing and clearance of beta-amyloid protein may contribute to the disease's development.

5. Tau Protein Abnormalities:
Tau protein abnormalities, such as the formation of tau tangles inside neurons, are another key pathological feature of Alzheimer's. These tangles disrupt neuronal function and contribute to cognitive decline.

6. Neuroinflammation:
Chronic neuroinflammation is observed in Alzheimer's. The brain's immune cells, microglia, become activated in response to beta-amyloid plaques and produce inflammatory molecules that can harm neurons.

7. Vascular Health:
Cardiovascular risk factors, including high blood pressure, high cholesterol, and diabetes, are associated with an increased risk of Alzheimer's disease. Poor vascular health can impair blood flow to the brain, potentially contributing to cognitive decline.

8. Lifestyle Factors:
Certain lifestyle choices can influence Alzheimer's risk. These include a diet high in saturated fats and low in antioxidants, lack of physical activity, smoking, and excessive alcohol consumption.

9. Traumatic Brain Injury (TBI):

A history of severe head injuries, particularly repeated concussions, is linked to a higher risk of developing Alzheimer's later in life.

10. Education and Cognitive Engagement:
Lower levels of education and limited cognitive engagement throughout life may be associated with a higher risk of Alzheimer's.

While these causes and risk factors provide insights into Alzheimer's disease, it's essential to recognize that the condition likely arises from a complex interplay of genetic, environmental, and lifestyle factors. Ongoing research aims to better understand these factors, paving the way for potential prevention and treatment strategies to combat this challenging neurodegenerative disease.

Genetic Factors

Genetic factors play a significant role in the development of Alzheimer's disease, influencing an individual's susceptibility to this complex neurodegenerative condition. While Alzheimer's is not solely determined by genetics, understanding the genetic components is crucial for identifying individuals at higher risk and advancing research in this field:

1. Early-Onset Familial Alzheimer's:
A small percentage of Alzheimer's cases, known as early-onset familial Alzheimer's disease (EOFAD), are directly linked to

genetic mutations. Mutations in specific genes, including Amyloid Precursor Protein (APP), Presenilin 1 (PSEN1), and Presenilin 2 (PSEN2), are associated with the development of Alzheimer's at a relatively young age (usually in one's 40s and 50s). These mutations affect the processing of amyloid beta protein and contribute to the formation of beta-amyloid plaques, a hallmark of the disease.

2. Late-Onset Alzheimer's and APOE Gene:
The majority of Alzheimer's cases fall into the late-onset category, which typically occurs after the age of 65. The most substantial genetic risk factor for late-onset Alzheimer's is the presence of the APOE ε4 allele of the apolipoprotein E (APOE) gene. Individuals who inherit one or two copies of the APOE ε4 allele have an increased risk of developing Alzheimer's and often experience an earlier onset of symptoms.

3. APOE ε2 and ε3 Alleles:
Conversely, the APOE ε2 allele is associated with a reduced risk of Alzheimer's, and individuals with this allele may develop the disease later in life. The APOE ε3 allele is considered neutral in terms of Alzheimer's risk. These alleles have different effects on the metabolism and clearance of beta-amyloid in the brain.

4. Polygenic Risk:
Late-onset Alzheimer's is a complex, multifactorial disease influenced by multiple genes. Researchers have identified several other genetic risk factors, often referred to as "polygenic risk," which contribute in combination to a person's overall risk. These risk factors involve various genes associated with processes like inflammation, cholesterol metabolism, and synaptic function.

5. Interaction with Environmental Factors:

It's important to note that while genetic factors significantly influence Alzheimer's risk, they do not guarantee the development of the disease. Interactions between genetic and environmental factors, such as lifestyle choices and cardiovascular health, also play a role in determining an individual's susceptibility.

Understanding genetic factors in Alzheimer's is crucial for early diagnosis, risk assessment, and the development of potential treatments. Ongoing research aims to uncover additional genetic markers and understand how these genes interact to better predict and ultimately prevent or treat this devastating condition.

Environmental Factors

Alzheimer's disease, a devastating neurodegenerative disorder, is influenced by various environmental factors that interact with genetic predispositions. While genetics plays a significant role in Alzheimer's, environmental factors are increasingly recognized as important contributors to the disease's development and progression.

One key environmental factor is lifestyle choices. Unhealthy habits such as a diet high in saturated fats and sugars, lack of physical activity, smoking, and excessive alcohol consumption have been associated with a higher risk of developing Alzheimer's. These factors can lead to conditions like obesity, diabetes, and hypertension, which increase the risk of cognitive decline.

Exposure to environmental toxins is another concern. Prolonged exposure to pollutants like heavy metals (e.g., lead and mercury), pesticides, and air pollution has been linked to cognitive impairments and an increased risk of Alzheimer's. These substances can accumulate in the brain and contribute to neuroinflammation and oxidative stress, both of which are implicated in Alzheimer's pathology.

Chronic stress is also considered an environmental risk factor. Prolonged stress can lead to elevated levels of stress hormones like cortisol, which may damage the brain's structure and function. This can promote the accumulation of beta-amyloid plaques and tau tangles, characteristic features of Alzheimer's disease.

Social and cognitive engagement can influence Alzheimer's risk as well. Individuals with rich social lives and mentally stimulating activities, such as reading or puzzles, tend to have a lower risk of cognitive decline. Engaging in meaningful social interactions and mental exercises may promote brain health and resilience against Alzheimer's.

Furthermore, traumatic brain injuries (TBIs) have gained attention as a significant environmental factor. A history of head injuries, particularly repetitive concussions, has been linked to an increased risk of Alzheimer's, possibly due to the disruption of brain structure and function.

In conclusion, environmental factors play a crucial role in the development and progression of Alzheimer's disease. While genetics is a key determinant, lifestyle choices, exposure to toxins, chronic stress, social engagement, and traumatic brain injuries can significantly influence an individual's susceptibility to the disease. Recognizing and addressing these environmental factors through healthier living and preventive measures is essential in the fight against Alzheimer's.

Lifestyle and Alzheimer's

Lifestyle choices play a pivotal role in the development and progression of Alzheimer's disease, a neurodegenerative disorder that affects millions of individuals worldwide. Research has increasingly highlighted the link between certain lifestyle factors and the risk of developing Alzheimer's, underscoring the importance of adopting a brain-healthy lifestyle.

Diet is a crucial aspect of lifestyle that can influence Alzheimer's risk. Consuming a diet rich in antioxidants, omega-3 fatty acids, and other nutrients found in fruits, vegetables, and fish has been associated with a reduced risk of cognitive decline. Conversely, diets high in saturated fats and refined sugars may contribute to inflammation and oxidative stress in the brain, which are linked to Alzheimer's pathology.

Physical activity is another significant lifestyle factor. Regular exercise not only promotes cardiovascular health but also enhances blood flow to the brain and stimulates the release of brain-derived neurotrophic factor (BDNF), a protein that supports the growth and maintenance of neurons. Engaging in aerobic and strength training exercises has been shown to reduce the risk of cognitive decline and may help delay the onset of Alzheimer's symptoms.

Mental stimulation and social engagement are essential for brain health. Activities such as reading, solving puzzles, learning new skills, and maintaining an active social life can help keep the brain sharp and resilient against Alzheimer's. These activities stimulate neural connections and may contribute to the growth of new brain cells.

Sleep patterns also impact cognitive function. Poor sleep quality and inadequate sleep duration have been linked to an increased risk of Alzheimer's. During sleep, the brain undergoes essential processes, such as the removal of toxic waste products like beta-amyloid, which is associated with Alzheimer's pathology. Prioritizing good sleep hygiene is crucial for maintaining brain health.

Managing stress is yet another lifestyle factor that can influence Alzheimer's risk. Chronic stress can lead to elevated levels of stress hormones, which may harm the brain and contribute to cognitive decline. Stress-reduction techniques like mindfulness meditation, yoga, and relaxation exercises can be beneficial in maintaining cognitive well-being.

In conclusion, lifestyle choices have a substantial impact on Alzheimer's disease. A brain-healthy lifestyle that includes a balanced diet, regular physical activity, mental stimulation, quality sleep, and stress management can help reduce the risk of cognitive decline and support overall brain health. By adopting these practices, individuals can take proactive steps toward minimizing their risk of developing Alzheimer's and promoting a higher quality of life as they age.

Chapter 4

The Pathology of Alzheimer's

Alzheimer's disease is a devastating neurodegenerative disorder that primarily affects the elderly population. It is characterized by progressive cognitive decline, memory loss, and impaired daily functioning. The pathology of Alzheimer's disease is complex and involves multiple mechanisms that lead to the accumulation of abnormal protein aggregates in the brain.

One of the hallmarks of Alzheimer's pathology is the presence of amyloid plaques. These plaques are composed of beta-amyloid protein fragments that clump together and accumulate in the spaces between nerve cells. This accumulation disrupts communication between neurons and is believed to be a key factor in the cognitive decline observed in Alzheimer's patients.

Another prominent feature of Alzheimer's pathology is the formation of neurofibrillary tangles. These tangles are composed of twisted and hyperphosphorylated tau protein, which is normally involved in maintaining the structural integrity of neurons. In Alzheimer's disease, tau protein becomes abnormally modified, leading to the formation of tangles inside neurons. This disrupts the internal structure of neurons and impairs their function.

In addition to amyloid plaques and neurofibrillary tangles, chronic inflammation in the brain, oxidative stress, and the loss of synaptic connections between neurons contribute to the pathology of Alzheimer's disease. The exact cause of Alzheimer's remains unclear, but genetic and environmental factors are thought to play a role in its development.

As the disease progresses, these pathological changes spread throughout the brain, causing widespread neuronal damage and cell death. This leads to a decline in cognitive function, memory loss, and eventually the inability to perform even basic daily tasks.

Understanding the pathology of Alzheimer's is crucial for developing effective treatments and interventions. Current research is focused on targeting amyloid plaques and tau tangles, as well as exploring inflammation and oxidative stress as potential therapeutic targets. While there is no cure for Alzheimer's disease yet, advances in our understanding of its pathology offer hope for the development of more effective treatments in the future.

Amyloid Plaques

Amyloid plaques play a central role in the pathology of Alzheimer's disease, a devastating neurodegenerative disorder that affects millions of individuals worldwide, primarily in older age. These plaques are one of the two hallmark pathological features of Alzheimer's, with the other being neurofibrillary tangles, and they contribute significantly to the cognitive decline and neuronal dysfunction observed in affected individuals.

Amyloid plaques consist primarily of beta-amyloid protein fragments that aggregate and accumulate in the extracellular spaces between nerve cells, or neurons, in the brain. These protein fragments are typically produced when a larger protein, called amyloid precursor protein (APP), is broken down. However, in Alzheimer's disease, there is an imbalance in the production and clearance of beta-amyloid, leading to the buildup of these toxic protein clumps.

The accumulation of amyloid plaques disrupts normal neuronal function in several ways. First, it interferes with synaptic transmission—the communication between neurons—by physically blocking the synapses. This disrupts the flow of electrical signals and impairs cognitive processes such as memory, reasoning, and problem-solving.

Furthermore, beta-amyloid is neurotoxic and can trigger inflammation in the brain, leading to further damage to neurons. This chronic inflammation contributes to the progressive nature of Alzheimer's disease and exacerbates the neuronal dysfunction and cell death associated with the condition.

Research into Alzheimer's disease has focused extensively on understanding the mechanisms behind the formation of amyloid plaques and finding ways to prevent or clear them. Potential treatments under investigation include drugs aimed at reducing the production of beta-amyloid, enhancing its clearance, or targeting the toxic effects of these plaques on neurons.

While amyloid plaques are a defining feature of Alzheimer's disease, it's important to note that they often coexist with neurofibrillary tangles composed of hyperphosphorylated tau protein. Together, these pathological changes lead to the devastating cognitive decline and loss of independence that characterize Alzheimer's disease. Understanding the role of amyloid plaques in Alzheimer's pathology is critical for the development of effective therapies and interventions to slow or halt the progression of this debilitating condition.

Tau Tangles

Tau tangles are a significant pathological feature of Alzheimer's disease, alongside amyloid plaques, and play a crucial role in the progression of this neurodegenerative disorder. These tangles are composed of abnormal accumulations of tau protein within neurons and are associated with widespread neuronal dysfunction and cognitive decline.

In healthy neurons, tau protein plays a vital role in stabilizing microtubules, which are essential for maintaining the cell's structural integrity and facilitating the transport of nutrients and other essential materials within the neuron. However, in Alzheimer's disease and related tauopathies, tau protein undergoes abnormal modifications, particularly hyperphosphorylation. This causes tau to detach from microtubules, preventing them from functioning correctly and leading to structural instability within neurons.

As tau proteins aggregate, they form twisted tangles within neurons, disrupting the normal cellular machinery and leading to cell death. These tangles are particularly prevalent in brain regions crucial for memory and cognitive function, such as the hippocampus and cortex. The presence of tau tangles correlates closely with the severity of cognitive impairment in Alzheimer's patients, making them a key pathological marker.

The spread of tau pathology follows a characteristic pattern in Alzheimer's disease, starting in specific brain regions and gradually spreading to others. This progression corresponds with the clinical stages of the disease, from mild cognitive impairment to advanced dementia.

Understanding the role of tau tangles in Alzheimer's disease has prompted extensive research efforts to develop therapies that target tau pathology. Potential treatments include drugs aimed at preventing tau phosphorylation, clearing abnormal tau aggregates, or stabilizing microtubules to counteract the toxic effects of tau tangles. These approaches are still in the experimental stage, and much work remains to be done to develop effective treatments for Alzheimer's disease.

In summary, tau tangles represent a critical pathological feature in Alzheimer's disease, contributing to neuronal dysfunction and cognitive decline. Research into the mechanisms of tau aggregation and the development of tau-targeted therapies offer hope for future treatments that can slow or potentially halt the progression of this devastating condition.

Other Biomarkers

In addition to amyloid plaques and tau tangles, several other biomarkers are emerging as valuable tools for diagnosing and understanding Alzheimer's disease. These biomarkers offer insights into different aspects of the disease, including its progression and potential causes. Here are some notable examples:

1. Cerebrospinal Fluid (CSF) Biomarkers: CSF analysis has revealed specific biomarkers associated with Alzheimer's disease. Increased levels of certain proteins, such as tau and phosphorylated tau (p-tau), and decreased levels of beta-amyloid in the CSF are indicative of Alzheimer's pathology. These biomarkers are useful for early detection and differential diagnosis.

2. Neuroimaging Biomarkers: Advanced neuroimaging techniques like positron emission tomography (PET) and magnetic resonance imaging (MRI) allow researchers and clinicians to visualize structural and functional changes in the brain. PET scans can detect amyloid plaques and tau tangles directly, while MRI can reveal brain atrophy patterns associated with Alzheimer's disease.

3. Blood-Based Biomarkers: Research is ongoing to identify blood-based biomarkers that can provide a less invasive and more accessible means of diagnosing Alzheimer's disease. Potential blood biomarkers include neurofilament light chain (NfL), which is associated with neuronal damage, and various proteins and metabolites associated with Alzheimer's pathology.

4. Genetic Biomarkers: Genetic factors play a significant role in Alzheimer's risk. Mutations in genes like APP, PSEN1, and PSEN2 are associated with familial Alzheimer's disease. Additionally, the APOE ε4 allele is a well-established genetic risk factor for late-onset Alzheimer's disease.

5. Inflammation Markers: Inflammation in the brain is thought to contribute to Alzheimer's pathology. Biomarkers associated with inflammation, such as cytokines and microglial activation markers,

are being studied to better understand the role of neuroinflammation in the disease.

6. Metabolic Biomarkers: Metabolic changes in the brain and body may be associated with Alzheimer's disease. Studies are exploring metabolic biomarkers, including those related to glucose metabolism and lipid profiles, to gain insights into the disease's metabolic aspects.

7. Epigenetic Biomarkers: Epigenetic changes, such as DNA methylation and histone modifications, may influence Alzheimer's risk and progression. Research into epigenetic biomarkers is uncovering potential links between these molecular modifications and the disease.

These biomarkers offer valuable insights into Alzheimer's disease, aiding in early diagnosis, monitoring disease progression, and identifying potential therapeutic targets. As research continues, the hope is that these biomarkers will contribute to the development of more accurate diagnostic tools and effective treatments for this challenging neurodegenerative disorder.

Chapter 5

Diagnosis and Early Detection

Diagnosing Alzheimer's disease and detecting it at an early stage are crucial for several reasons. Early intervention can help patients and their families plan for the future, access appropriate medical and social support, and potentially slow the progression of the disease through early treatment and lifestyle changes. Diagnosing Alzheimer's disease typically involves a multi-faceted approach:

1. Clinical Evaluation: Physicians often begin with a thorough clinical evaluation, including medical history, cognitive assessments, and neurological exams. They may interview the patient and their family members to understand the onset and progression of cognitive symptoms.

2. Cognitive Tests: Standardized cognitive tests, such as the Mini-Mental State Examination (MMSE) or the Montreal Cognitive Assessment (MoCA), are administered to assess memory, language, problem-solving, and other cognitive functions.

3. Neuroimaging:Brain imaging techniques like MRI and PET scans can reveal structural and functional changes in the brain. MRI can show atrophy patterns, while PET scans can detect the presence of amyloid plaques and tau tangles.

4. Cerebrospinal Fluid Analysis:A lumbar puncture can be performed to analyze cerebrospinal fluid for biomarkers like beta-amyloid and tau proteins, which are indicative of Alzheimer's pathology.

5. Genetic Testing: In some cases, genetic testing may be considered, especially when there is a family history of early-onset Alzheimer's disease or known genetic mutations associated with the condition.

Early detection of Alzheimer's often relies on the combination of these methods. However, challenges remain in accurately diagnosing the disease in its early stages, as many of the cognitive symptoms can overlap with normal aging or other neurological conditions.

Advancements in research are continually improving early detection methods. Blood-based biomarkers, for instance, are being explored as less invasive and more accessible tools for identifying individuals at risk for Alzheimer's. Additionally, machine learning and artificial intelligence are being employed to analyze large datasets of cognitive assessments, imaging, and biomarker data to improve diagnostic accuracy and predict the risk of developing Alzheimer's.

Efforts to detect Alzheimer's disease in its preclinical or prodromal stages, even before noticeable cognitive symptoms occur, hold promise for future interventions. Early detection and diagnosis remain essential for the development of effective treatments and support systems to alleviate the burden of Alzheimer's disease on patients, caregivers, and society as a whole.

Recognizing the Signs

Recognizing the signs of Alzheimer's disease is crucial for early intervention and providing appropriate care and support to affected individuals. Alzheimer's is a progressive neurodegenerative disorder that primarily affects memory and cognitive function. Here are some key signs and symptoms to watch for:

1. **Memory Loss:** One of the most common early signs is significant memory loss, especially in recent events or conversations. Individuals may repeatedly ask the same questions or forget important dates and events.

2. **Difficulty with Familiar Tasks:** People with Alzheimer's may struggle to complete routine tasks they once handled with ease, such as cooking, managing finances, or following a familiar recipe.

3. **Disorientation:** Individuals may become disoriented in familiar places, forget where they are, or get lost in their own neighborhood. They may also lose track of time.

4. **Language Problems:** Alzheimer's can affect language skills, leading to difficulty finding the right words, repeating phrases, or struggling to follow or join in conversations.

5. **Poor Judgment:** Impaired judgment and decision-making are common. This can manifest in reckless financial choices, neglect of personal hygiene, or poor judgment regarding safety.

6. **Misplacing Items:** People with Alzheimer's often misplace objects and struggle to retrace their steps to find them. They may put items in unusual places, such as keys in the refrigerator.

7. **Changes in Personality and Mood:** Alzheimer's can lead to mood swings, irritability, depression, and anxiety. Personality changes, such as becoming more withdrawn or suspicious, may also occur.

8. **Loss of Initiative:** Individuals may lose interest in activities they once enjoyed, become passive, or avoid social interactions and hobbies.

9. **Difficulty with Visual and Spatial Abilities:** Problems with depth perception, judging distances, and recognizing familiar faces or objects can develop.

10. **Difficulty with Problem-Solving:** Complex tasks that involve planning and problem-solving become increasingly challenging.

Recognizing these signs is essential, but it's important to note that Alzheimer's disease progresses differently in each individual. Not everyone will experience all of these symptoms, and they may manifest at different rates.

If you or a loved one notice these signs or are concerned about memory and cognitive changes, it's crucial to seek a comprehensive medical evaluation from a healthcare professional. Early diagnosis allows for appropriate interventions, treatment, and support services, which can help manage the condition more effectively and improve the quality of life for individuals living with Alzheimer's and their caregivers.

Common Symptoms

Alzheimer's disease is a progressive neurodegenerative disorder that primarily affects cognitive function. While the disease can manifest differently in each individual, there are common symptoms that characterize Alzheimer's as it progresses through its various stages. These symptoms often become more intense over time:

1. **Memory Loss:** Difficulty remembering recent events, names, and important dates is one of the hallmark symptoms of Alzheimer's. Individuals may forget conversations, appointments, or where they placed everyday items like keys or eyeglasses.

2. **Disorientation and Confusion:** People with Alzheimer's frequently become disoriented, forgetting the current date, time, or

their location. They may even lose track of seasons or the passage of time.

3. **Language Problems:** Individuals may struggle to find the right words, repeat themselves, or have difficulty following or participating in conversations. They may also have trouble understanding written or spoken language.

4. **Impaired Judgment:** Poor decision-making and impaired judgment are common, leading to issues like neglecting personal hygiene, falling for scams, or making unsafe choices.

5. **Difficulty with Problem-Solving:** Complex tasks that involve planning, organizing, or problem-solving become increasingly challenging. Managing finances, following recipes, or completing familiar tasks may become difficult.

6. **Personality Changes:** Alzheimer's can bring about personality changes, including mood swings, irritability, anxiety, and depression. Individuals may become more withdrawn or exhibit suspicious behavior.

7. **Loss of Initiative:** Apathy and a reduced interest in once-enjoyed activities are common. Individuals may become passive and show a lack of initiative in social or leisure activities.

8. **Visual and Spatial Problems:** Alzheimer's can affect visual and spatial abilities, leading to difficulty reading, judging distances, and recognizing familiar objects or faces.

9. **Misplacing Items:** Individuals often misplace objects and struggle to retrace their steps to find them. They may put items in unusual places, like putting shoes in the refrigerator.

10. **Difficulty with Familiar Tasks:** Routine tasks, such as cooking, dressing, or using household appliances, become progressively challenging as Alzheimer's advances.

11. **Social Withdrawal:** Many individuals with Alzheimer's gradually withdraw from social activities, hobbies, and interactions, often due to the difficulties they experience in communication and memory.

It's important to note that Alzheimer's progresses differently in each person, and the severity and timing of these symptoms can vary. In the early stages, these changes may be subtle and attributed to normal aging. However, as the disease advances, they become more pronounced and interfere with daily life.

Recognizing these common symptoms is crucial for early diagnosis and intervention, as early treatment and support can help manage the condition more effectively and improve the quality of life for both individuals living with Alzheimer's and their caregivers. If you or a loved one experience these symptoms, seeking a comprehensive medical evaluation is essential for an accurate diagnosis and appropriate care planning.

Stages of Alzheimer's

Alzheimer's disease is a progressive neurodegenerative disorder that typically unfolds in distinct stages, each marked by specific cognitive and functional changes. While the progression varies from person to person, these stages provide a general framework for understanding the course of the disease:

1. **Preclinical Stage:** Alzheimer's often begins with a preclinical phase, which can last for several years or even decades before noticeable symptoms emerge. During this stage, changes are occurring in the brain, such as the accumulation of abnormal proteins like beta-amyloid. However, individuals do not yet exhibit cognitive or functional deficits.

2. **Mild Cognitive Impairment (MCI):** The earliest recognizable stage of Alzheimer's is often characterized by mild cognitive impairment. Memory lapses, difficulty finding words, and challenges with planning or organization become apparent. Importantly, these cognitive changes are noticeable to the individual and their loved ones but do not yet significantly interfere with daily life.

3. **Early-Stage Alzheimer's:** As the disease progresses, the individual enters the early stage of Alzheimer's. In this stage, cognitive symptoms become more pronounced, affecting memory, language, and problem-solving abilities. Individuals may experience disorientation, difficulty managing finances, and a decline in their ability to work or engage in hobbies.

4. **Middle-Stage Alzheimer's:** The middle stage is marked by a more severe decline in cognitive and functional abilities. Individuals may struggle with basic tasks like dressing, bathing, and eating. Personality changes, agitation, and wandering behavior can also occur. Communication becomes increasingly challenging, and individuals may require assistance with daily activities.

5. **Late-Stage Alzheimer's:** In the final stage of the disease, individuals are profoundly impaired both cognitively and functionally. They often lose the ability to recognize loved ones, communicate verbally, or control bodily functions. Assistance with all aspects of daily life, including eating, mobility, and personal care, is necessary.

It's important to note that the duration of each stage can vary widely among individuals, with some progressing through the stages more rapidly than others. Additionally, not all individuals with Alzheimer's will experience every symptom associated with each stage.

Care and support requirements evolve with the progression of the disease. In the earlier stages, individuals may benefit from medication and cognitive therapies that can temporarily slow cognitive decline and improve quality of life. In the later stages, specialized care in a supportive environment becomes essential to ensure safety and comfort.

Understanding the stages of Alzheimer's is crucial for individuals, families, and caregivers to plan for the future, access appropriate resources, and provide the best possible care for those affected by this challenging and devastating condition

Chapter 6

The Diagnostic Process

The diagnostic process for Alzheimer's disease is a thorough and multi-step evaluation conducted by healthcare professionals to assess cognitive decline and rule out other potential causes. Here's an overview of the process involved:

1. **Clinical Assessment:** The process often begins with a comprehensive clinical assessment. A healthcare provider, typically a neurologist or geriatrician, interviews the individual and their family members to gather information about medical history, cognitive symptoms, and daily functioning.

2. **Cognitive Testing:** Standardized cognitive tests, such as the Mini-Mental State Examination (MMSE) or the Montreal Cognitive Assessment (MoCA), are administered to assess memory, language, reasoning, and other cognitive functions.

3. **Neuroimaging:** Brain imaging techniques like MRI or PET scans are used to visualize structural and functional changes in the brain. These scans can help rule out other conditions that may be causing cognitive symptoms and can sometimes detect hallmark signs of Alzheimer's, such as amyloid plaques and tau tangles.

4. **Laboratory Tests:** Blood tests may be conducted to rule out other medical conditions, such as thyroid dysfunction or vitamin deficiencies, that can mimic cognitive decline.

5. **Cerebrospinal Fluid Analysis:** In some cases, a lumbar puncture may be performed to analyze cerebrospinal fluid for biomarkers associated with Alzheimer's disease, such as elevated levels of tau and beta-amyloid proteins.

6. **Genetic Testing:** Genetic testing may be considered, especially in cases of early-onset Alzheimer's or when there is a family history of the disease. Certain genetic mutations are associated with a higher risk of developing Alzheimer's.

7. **Assessment of Functional Abilities:** Evaluating the individual's ability to perform daily activities, such as cooking, managing finances, or dressing, is crucial in assessing functional impairment.

8. **Longitudinal Observation:** Sometimes, the diagnostic process involves monitoring cognitive changes over time to establish a pattern of decline consistent with Alzheimer's.

A conclusive Alzheimer's diagnosis is typically made when other potential causes of cognitive decline have been ruled out, and cognitive testing and biomarker assessments suggest the presence of Alzheimer's pathology. Early diagnosis is essential for accessing appropriate care, interventions, and support services, as well as participating in clinical trials for potential treatments. It allows individuals and their families to plan for the future and make informed decisions about their care.

Medical Evaluation

A medical evaluation for Alzheimer's disease is a comprehensive process aimed at diagnosing the condition, understanding its severity, ruling out other potential causes of cognitive impairment, and developing an appropriate care and treatment plan. Here's an in-depth look at the key components of a medical evaluation for Alzheimer's:

1. **Clinical Assessment:** The evaluation typically begins with a thorough clinical assessment conducted by a healthcare professional, often a neurologist or geriatrician. This involves taking a detailed medical history, including any family history of

Alzheimer's or related disorders. The healthcare provider interviews the individual and their family members to gather information about cognitive symptoms, changes in daily functioning, and any accompanying behavioral or mood changes.

2. **Cognitive Testing:** Standardized cognitive tests are administered to assess various aspects of cognitive function, including memory, language, attention, and problem-solving abilities. Tests like the Mini-Mental State Examination (MMSE) and the Montreal Cognitive Assessment (MoCA) are commonly used.

3. **Neuroimaging:** Brain imaging techniques such as magnetic resonance imaging (MRI) and positron emission tomography (PET) scans are employed to visualize structural and functional changes in the brain. These scans can help detect brain atrophy, rule out other conditions, and sometimes reveal the presence of Alzheimer's-specific abnormalities, like amyloid plaques and tau tangles.

4. **Laboratory Tests:** Blood tests may be conducted to identify or rule out other potential causes of cognitive impairment, such as thyroid dysfunction, vitamin deficiencies, or infections. These tests help ensure that the cognitive symptoms are not due to a reversible or treatable condition.

5. **Cerebrospinal Fluid Analysis:** In some cases, a lumbar puncture may be performed to analyze cerebrospinal fluid for biomarkers associated with Alzheimer's, such as elevated levels of tau and beta-amyloid proteins. This can provide additional evidence of Alzheimer's pathology.

6. **Genetic Testing:** Genetic testing may be considered, especially if there is a family history of Alzheimer's or when early-

onset Alzheimer's is suspected. Certain genetic mutations are associated with a higher risk of developing the disease.

7. **Functional Assessment:** Evaluating the individual's ability to perform daily activities and instrumental activities of daily living (ADLs and IADLs) is critical for assessing functional impairment and determining the level of support and care required.

8. **Psychological and Behavioral Assessment:** Assessing changes in mood, behavior, and psychiatric symptoms, such as depression and anxiety, is essential, as these can be part of the clinical picture in Alzheimer's.

A medical evaluation for Alzheimer's is a meticulous and often multi-disciplinary process that helps healthcare providers make an accurate diagnosis, stage the disease, and develop a comprehensive care plan. An early and accurate diagnosis is crucial for accessing appropriate treatments, interventions, and support services that can enhance the quality of life for individuals with Alzheimer's and their caregivers.

Cognitive Testing

Cognitive testing is a fundamental component of the diagnostic process for Alzheimer's disease and other forms of cognitive impairment. These tests are designed to assess an individual's cognitive abilities, including memory, attention, language, reasoning, and problem-solving skills. In the context of Alzheimer's, cognitive testing serves several important purposes:

1. **Early Detection:** Cognitive tests can help identify subtle cognitive changes that may be indicative of Alzheimer's disease, even in its earliest stages. Detecting these changes allows for timely intervention and treatment.

2. **Diagnosis Confirmation:** When combined with other clinical assessments and biomarker testing, cognitive testing helps confirm an Alzheimer's diagnosis by providing objective evidence of cognitive impairment beyond what would be expected due to normal aging.

3. **Disease Staging:** Cognitive testing helps healthcare professionals assess the severity and progression of Alzheimer's disease. It allows them to categorize individuals into stages ranging from mild cognitive impairment (MCI) to moderate and severe Alzheimer's.

4. **Treatment Planning:** Cognitive tests provide a baseline of cognitive function, enabling healthcare providers to track changes over time. This information is invaluable for tailoring treatment plans and interventions to the individual's specific needs.

5. **Monitoring Response to Treatment:** For those receiving Alzheimer's medications or participating in clinical trials, cognitive testing is a crucial tool for evaluating whether treatments are effectively slowing cognitive decline or improving cognitive function.

Common cognitive tests used in Alzheimer's diagnosis and monitoring include:

- **Mini-Mental State Examination (MMSE):** This widely used test assesses various cognitive functions, including orientation, memory, attention, language, and visuospatial abilities.

- **Montreal Cognitive Assessment (MoCA):** Similar to the MMSE, the MoCA assesses a broader range of cognitive functions, including executive function and abstract reasoning.

- **Alzheimer's Disease Assessment Scale-Cognitive Subscale (ADAS-Cog):** This test is often used in clinical trials and research settings to assess cognitive changes related to Alzheimer's disease.

- **Clock Drawing Test:** Individuals are asked to draw a clock face, set to a specific time. This test evaluates visuospatial abilities and executive function.

- **Verbal Memory Tests:** These tests assess an individual's ability to remember and recall words or short stories, which can be particularly useful for detecting memory deficits.

Cognitive testing is just one piece of the diagnostic puzzle for Alzheimer's, and it is often combined with other assessments, such as neurological exams, imaging studies, and biomarker testing, to provide a comprehensive evaluation. Early and accurate cognitive testing is essential for timely diagnosis and intervention, helping individuals and their families plan for the future and access appropriate care and support services.

Imaging and Biomarkers

Imaging and biomarkers are critical tools in the diagnosis, staging, and research of Alzheimer's disease. They provide valuable insights into the underlying pathology and progression of the disease, aiding in early detection and treatment monitoring. Here's an overview of their roles in Alzheimer's research and clinical practice:

Imaging Techniques:

1. **Magnetic Resonance Imaging (MRI):** MRI is commonly used to create detailed images of the brain's structure. It can reveal brain atrophy, which is often seen in Alzheimer's patients, especially in regions associated with memory and cognition.

2. **Positron Emission Tomography (PET):** PET scans can detect changes in brain metabolism and the accumulation of abnormal proteins like beta-amyloid and tau. Amyloid PET scans, in particular, can visualize the presence of amyloid plaques, a hallmark of Alzheimer's pathology.

3. **Functional MRI (fMRI):** fMRI measures changes in blood flow and can assess brain activity during cognitive tasks. It helps researchers understand how brain function is altered in Alzheimer's and can aid in early diagnosis by identifying functional changes before significant structural damage occurs.

Biomarkers

1. **Beta-Amyloid and Tau Proteins:** Biomarkers in cerebrospinal fluid (CSF) or blood can indicate the presence and accumulation of beta-amyloid and tau proteins. Elevated levels of

these proteins are associated with Alzheimer's pathology. CSF analysis can provide direct insights into the disease process.

2. **Neurofilament Light Chain (NfL):** Elevated levels of NfL in CSF or blood can indicate neuronal damage, which occurs in Alzheimer's and other neurodegenerative conditions. NfL is a promising biomarker for monitoring disease progression and response to treatment.

3. **Imaging Biomarkers:** In addition to visualizing amyloid plaques and tau tangles, PET scans can measure the binding of specific tracers to these proteins. Changes in binding patterns over time can help assess disease progression and treatment efficacy.

4. **Genetic Biomarkers:** Certain genetic factors, such as the APOE ε4 allele, are associated with an increased risk of developing Alzheimer's disease. Genetic testing can identify individuals at higher risk and inform early intervention strategies.

These imaging and biomarker techniques are not only valuable for diagnosis but also for ongoing research into Alzheimer's disease. They enable researchers to better understand the disease's mechanisms, track its progression, and evaluate the effectiveness of potential treatments in clinical trials. Additionally, advances in technology and research are continually improving the accuracy and accessibility of these diagnostic tools, offering hope for earlier and more precise Alzheimer's detection and intervention.

Chapter 7

Early Intervention

Early intervention in Alzheimer's disease is crucial for several reasons, primarily focused on improving the quality of life for affected individuals and their caregivers. While there is currently no cure for Alzheimer's, early diagnosis and intervention can significantly impact the course of the disease and provide various benefits:

1. **Access to Treatment:** Early diagnosis allows individuals to receive available medications, such as cholinesterase inhibitors and memantine, that can temporarily alleviate cognitive symptoms and improve daily functioning. These treatments are most effective when initiated in the early stages of the disease.

2. **Participation in Clinical Trials:** Early intervention provides individuals the opportunity to participate in clinical trials for experimental treatments and therapies. These trials aim to develop new medications and interventions that may slow or halt the progression of Alzheimer's.

3. **Disease Management:** Early intervention allows individuals and their families to proactively plan for the future. They can make informed decisions about care, legal and financial matters, and long-term care options while the individual is still able to participate in these discussions.

4. **Lifestyle Modifications:** Early diagnosis enables individuals to make lifestyle changes that may help slow cognitive decline.

These changes include adopting a brain-healthy diet, engaging in regular physical and mental exercise, managing chronic conditions, and staying socially and cognitively active.

5. **Support Services:** Early intervention provides access to support services and resources that can enhance the quality of life for both individuals with Alzheimer's and their caregivers. Support groups, respite care, and education programs can help caregivers better navigate the challenges of caring for a loved one with Alzheimer's.

6. **Improved Safety:** Cognitive changes in Alzheimer's can increase the risk of accidents and wandering. Early intervention allows families to implement safety measures, such as home modifications and tracking devices, to protect the individual with Alzheimer's.

7. **Reduced Caregiver Stress:** Early intervention can help caregivers better understand the disease and learn coping strategies. Reducing caregiver stress and burnout is essential for maintaining the health and well-being of both caregivers and individuals with Alzheimer's.

8. **Enhanced Emotional Well-Being:** Early intervention and appropriate treatment can help manage behavioral and psychological symptoms of Alzheimer's, such as depression, anxiety, and agitation, leading to an improved overall emotional state for the individual.

In conclusion, early intervention in Alzheimer's disease is not about finding a cure but about optimizing the individual's quality of life, providing access to available treatments and support services, and allowing for informed planning for the future. It empowers individuals and their families to navigate the challenges of Alzheimer's with greater resilience and hope.

Medications and Treatments

Medications and treatments for Alzheimer's disease aim to alleviate symptoms, slow disease progression, and improve the quality of life for affected individuals. While there is no cure for Alzheimer's, several medications and non-pharmacological interventions are available to address various aspects of the disease:

1. Cholinesterase Inhibitors: These drugs, including donepezil (Aricept), rivastigmine (Exelon), and galantamine (Razadyne), work by boosting levels of acetylcholine, a neurotransmitter involved in memory and cognition. Cholinesterase inhibitors can temporarily improve cognitive function and daily living activities, especially in the early and mild stages of Alzheimer's.

2. Memantine: Memantine (Namenda) is an N-methyl-D-aspartate (NMDA) receptor antagonist that helps regulate glutamate, another neurotransmitter. It is often prescribed in moderate to severe Alzheimer's to manage cognitive symptoms, including memory, language, and reasoning.

3. Combination Therapy: Some individuals with Alzheimer's may benefit from a combination of cholinesterase inhibitors and memantine to target multiple aspects of the disease.

4. Antipsychotic Medications: In cases of severe agitation, aggression, or psychosis in Alzheimer's patients, antipsychotic medications may be prescribed, but their use is carefully monitored due to potential side effects.

5. Behavioral and Psychosocial Interventions: Non-pharmacological interventions are vital in managing Alzheimer's symptoms. These include cognitive stimulation therapy, occupational therapy, and psychosocial support programs. These interventions aim to enhance cognitive function, provide emotional support, and improve the individual's overall quality of life.

6. Lifestyle Modifications: Encouraging a brain-healthy lifestyle can help slow cognitive decline. This includes regular physical exercise, a balanced diet rich in antioxidants and omega-3 fatty acids, social engagement, and cognitive stimulation through activities like puzzles and games.

7. Clinical Trials: Participation in clinical trials can provide access to experimental treatments and therapies aimed at slowing or halting the progression of Alzheimer's disease. These trials often test new medications, vaccines, or interventions designed to target the underlying pathology.

It's important to note that the effectiveness of these medications and treatments can vary from person to person, and they may have limited impact on the advanced stages of the disease. Early diagnosis and intervention tend to yield better results. Healthcare providers work closely with individuals and their families to tailor treatment plans to individual needs, monitor medication efficacy, and adjust treatments as the disease progresses.

While there is no cure for Alzheimer's, ongoing research holds promise for more effective treatments and interventions in the future. In the meantime, the goal of current treatments is to enhance the well-being and functional abilities of individuals with

Alzheimer's, allowing them to live as independently and comfortably as possible.

Lifestyle Modifications

Lifestyle modifications are an essential component of managing Alzheimer's disease. While there is no cure for this neurodegenerative condition, adopting certain lifestyle changes can help improve the quality of life for individuals with Alzheimer's and may even slow the progression of the disease. Here are key lifestyle modifications:

1. **Physical Exercise:** Regular physical activity is beneficial for both physical and cognitive health. Exercise improves blood flow to the brain, reduces inflammation, and stimulates the release of chemicals that promote brain cell growth. Aerobic exercises like walking, swimming, and dancing are particularly effective.

2. **Brain-Healthy Diet:** A well-balanced diet can support brain health. Diets rich in antioxidants (found in fruits and vegetables), omega-3 fatty acids (found in fish), and low in saturated fats can help reduce the risk of cognitive decline. Staying hydrated is also important.

3. **Social Engagement:** Staying socially active is crucial for maintaining cognitive function. Engaging in social activities, such as group outings, clubs, or classes, can help stimulate the brain and improve mood.

4. **Cognitive Stimulation:** Keeping the mind active through activities like puzzles, crossword puzzles, reading, and learning new skills can help maintain cognitive function. Cognitive stimulation therapy is specifically designed to engage individuals with Alzheimer's in mental exercises.

5. **Sleep Management:** Quality sleep is essential for overall health and cognitive function. Establishing a regular sleep schedule and creating a comfortable sleep environment can improve sleep quality.

6. **Stress Reduction:** Chronic stress can have a negative impact on cognitive health. Stress-reduction techniques, such as mindfulness meditation, deep breathing exercises, and relaxation therapies, can help manage stress.

7. **Safety Precautions:** Implementing safety measures at home, such as removing tripping hazards, installing handrails, and using locks or alarms on doors and windows, can prevent accidents and promote independence.

8. **Medication Management:** Careful management of medications is essential, as medication side effects or interactions can affect cognitive function. Ensuring that medications are taken as prescribed and regularly reviewed by healthcare providers is crucial.

9. **Support System:** Building a strong support system, which may include family, friends, and support groups, can help both individuals with Alzheimer's and their caregivers cope with the challenges of the disease.

10. **Legal and Financial Planning:** Early planning for legal and financial matters, including power of attorney and advance

directives, can provide clarity and peace of mind for both individuals with Alzheimer's and their families.

It's important to note that while these lifestyle modifications can contribute to a better quality of life and potentially slow cognitive decline, they are not a substitute for medical treatment and care. Individuals with Alzheimer's should work closely with healthcare providers to develop a comprehensive care plan that includes medication management, regular medical evaluations, and support services tailored to their needs.

Support for Caregivers

Support for caregivers of individuals with Alzheimer's disease is essential, as caring for a loved one with this progressive condition can be physically, emotionally, and mentally challenging. Caregivers often face a significant burden, and accessing the right support is crucial to ensure the well-being of both the caregiver and the person with Alzheimer's. Here are some key forms of support for caregivers:

1. **Education and Information:** Caregivers benefit from understanding Alzheimer's disease and its progression. Educational resources, workshops, and informational materials can help caregivers develop strategies for managing symptoms and providing appropriate care.

2. **Support Groups:** Support groups provide a safe space for caregivers to connect with others facing similar challenges. These groups offer emotional support, practical advice, and a sense of community where caregivers can share experiences and coping strategies.

3. **Respite Care:** Respite care services allow caregivers to take short breaks from their caregiving responsibilities. These breaks are essential for preventing burnout and maintaining the caregiver's own health and well-being.

4. **Professional Help:** Access to healthcare professionals, such as geriatric care managers and social workers, can assist caregivers in navigating the complexities of Alzheimer's care, coordinating medical appointments, and accessing available resources.

5. **In-Home Services:** Various in-home services, such as home health aides, can assist with daily tasks like bathing, dressing, and meal preparation. This support allows caregivers to focus on other aspects of caregiving and self-care.

6. **Adult Day Care Programs:** Adult day care centers offer a structured environment for individuals with Alzheimer's, providing social interaction and cognitive stimulation while caregivers attend to other responsibilities.

7. **Legal and Financial Assistance:** Caregivers may need legal guidance for setting up power of attorney or addressing financial matters. Legal and financial professionals with expertise in elder law can be invaluable.

8. **Technology and Apps:** There are numerous apps and technologies designed to support caregivers, from medication management apps to GPS trackers that help locate individuals who may wander due to Alzheimer's-related confusion.

9. **Community Resources:** Many communities offer services and programs specifically designed to support Alzheimer's

caregivers. These resources can include transportation assistance, meal delivery, and adult day programs.

10. **Emotional Support:** Caregivers often experience feelings of stress, guilt, and grief. Access to counseling, therapy, or support services focused on emotional well-being can help caregivers cope with these complex emotions.

Recognizing the needs of caregivers is essential, and their well-being directly impacts the quality of care they can provide to their loved ones with Alzheimer's. A strong support network, including family, friends, and professional assistance, is key to ensuring that caregivers can provide the best possible care while also taking care of their own health and emotional needs.

Chapter 8

Living with Alzheimer's

Living with Alzheimer's disease is a complex journey that presents unique challenges for both individuals diagnosed with the condition and their families. Alzheimer's is a progressive neurodegenerative disease that affects memory, cognition, and daily functioning. While it poses significant challenges, it's important to recognize that people with Alzheimer's can still lead meaningful and fulfilling lives, especially with appropriate support and adjustments. Here are some key aspects of living with Alzheimer's:

1. **Early Diagnosis:** Early diagnosis is critical for individuals with Alzheimer's, as it allows them to access treatments, interventions, and support services that can help manage symptoms and improve quality of life.

2. **Coping Strategies:** Learning and implementing coping strategies can make a significant difference in daily life. These strategies may involve memory aids, routines, and techniques to manage forgetfulness and confusion.

3. **Support Networks:** Building a strong support network of family, friends, and healthcare professionals is essential. Loved

ones and caregivers play a vital role in providing emotional and practical support throughout the journey.

4. **Staying Engaged:** Staying socially and mentally engaged can help individuals with Alzheimer's maintain cognitive function and emotional well-being. Engaging in activities they enjoy, participating in support groups, and pursuing hobbies can be beneficial.

5. **Medication Management:** Medications prescribed by healthcare providers can help manage cognitive symptoms and behavioral changes associated with Alzheimer's. Regular monitoring and adjustment of medications are often necessary.

6. **Safety Measures:** Safety at home is a significant concern. Taking steps to reduce hazards, such as installing handrails and alarms, can prevent accidents and ensure a safe living environment.

7. **Legal and Financial Planning:** Early legal and financial planning, including power of attorney and advance directives, allows individuals to make important decisions about their future care and financial matters while they are still capable.

8. **Emotional Well-Being:** Emotional support is crucial for individuals with Alzheimer's. They may experience frustration, anxiety, and depression. Seeking emotional support through counseling, therapy, or support groups can help manage these feelings.

9. **Caregiver Relationships:** Alzheimer's often places a significant burden on caregivers. Open communication, respite care, and seeking caregiver support are essential for maintaining

caregiver well-being and ensuring quality care for the individual with Alzheimer's.

10. **Advocacy and Awareness:** Many individuals with Alzheimer's become advocates, raising awareness about the disease and participating in research studies or clinical trials to contribute to the search for a cure or more effective treatments.

Living with Alzheimer's requires adaptation and support, and while it presents challenges, it's possible to find moments of joy, connection, and fulfillment throughout the journey. With the right resources and a supportive community, individuals with Alzheimer's and their families can navigate this challenging path with resilience and grace.

Navigating Care Options

Navigating care options for Alzheimer's disease can be a complex and emotionally challenging process. As the disease increases individuals with Alzheimer's normally require increasing stages of care and support. Here's an overview of the care options available and important considerations for families:

1. **Home Care:** Many families start by providing care at home. This can include family members assisting with daily activities, hiring home health aides, and making home modifications to ensure safety. It's essential to assess the caregiver's ability to provide care and to consider respite care options to prevent caregiver burnout.

2. **Adult Day Care:** Adult day care centers offer structured programs and supervision during the day, allowing caregivers to

work or take a break. These programs can provide social engagement and cognitive stimulation for individuals with Alzheimer's.

3. **Assisted Living Facilities:** Assisted living facilities provide a level of care between independent living and skilled nursing care. They offer assistance with activities of daily living (ADLs) while promoting independence. Some facilities have specialized memory care units designed for individuals with Alzheimer's.

4. **Memory Care Units:** Memory care units within assisted living or skilled nursing facilities are specifically designed to cater to the unique needs of individuals with Alzheimer's. Staff members are trained to provide specialized care and engage residents in appropriate activities.

5. **Skilled Nursing Facilities (Nursing Homes):** Skilled nursing facilities offer 24-hour medical care and supervision. They are typically recommended for individuals in the advanced stages of Alzheimer's or those with complex medical needs.

6. **In-Home Hospice Care:** Hospice care focuses on providing comfort and support to individuals with advanced Alzheimer's. It is often chosen when curative treatments are no longer effective or appropriate.

Important considerations when navigating care options:

- **Assessment and Planning:** A comprehensive assessment by a healthcare provider can help determine the level of care needed. Developing a care plan that addresses the individual's unique needs is crucial.

- **Costs and Financial Planning:** Understand the costs associated with different care options and explore financial resources such as long-term care insurance, Medicare, Medicaid, and veterans' benefits.

- **Quality of Care:** Research and visit care facilities or providers to assess the quality of care, staff training, and the suitability of the environment for individuals with Alzheimer's.

- **Legal and Ethical Considerations:** Ensure that legal and ethical matters, such as advance directives and power of attorney, are addressed to make decisions in the best interests of the individual with Alzheimer's.

- **Family Communication:** Open and ongoing communication among family members is vital when making decisions about care options. Everyone should have a clear understanding of roles and responsibilities.

- **Regular Reassessment:** Care needs can change over time, so it's essential to regularly reassess the chosen care arrangement to ensure that it continues to meet the individual's needs.

Navigating care options for Alzheimer's requires careful planning, consideration of the individual's preferences, and a commitment to ensuring their safety and well-being throughout the progression of the disease. Consulting with healthcare professionals and seeking support from Alzheimer's associations and support groups can provide valuable guidance during this challenging journey.

Home Care vs. Assisted Living

 Choosing between home care and assisted living for an individual with Alzheimer's disease is a significant decision that depends on various factors, including the individual's needs, the family's preferences, and available resources. Both options have their advantages and drawbacks, and making the important choice wich requires careful consideration.

Home Care:

1. **Familiar Environment:** One of the most significant advantages of home care is that the individual can remain in a familiar environment, which can be comforting and less disorienting for someone with Alzheimer's.

2. **Individualized Care:** Home care allows for highly personalized care plans tailored to the specific needs of the individual. Family members can closely monitor the quality of care provided.

3. **Family Involvement:** Family members can be directly involved in caregiving, which can provide emotional support and strengthen relationships.

4. **Flexible Scheduling:** Home care allows for flexibility in scheduling care services, making it easier to adapt to the changing needs of the individual.

However, home care also has its challenges:

1. **Caregiver Burnout:** Providing care at home can be physically and emotionally demanding, leading to caregiver burnout if not properly managed. Respite care and support are essential.

2. **Safety Concerns:** Home environments may need modifications to ensure safety, such as installing locks on doors or removing tripping hazards.

3. **Limited Social Interaction:** Individuals receiving home care may have limited social interaction compared to those in assisted living settings, which could lead to feelings of isolation.

Assisted Living:

1. **Specialized Care:** Assisted living facilities often have memory care units staffed by professionals trained in Alzheimer's care. They can provide specialized support and activities tailored to the needs of individuals with Alzheimer's.

2. **Safety and Supervision:** Assisted living facilities are designed to be safe, minimizing risks of accidents or wandering. Trained staff can provide 24/7 supervision.

3. **Social Engagement:** Assisted living offers social opportunities and interactions with peers, which can be beneficial for individuals with Alzheimer's.

However here are some disadvantages to assisted living:

1. **Adjustment Period:** Moving to a new environment can be disorienting and emotionally challenging for the individual with Alzheimer's.

2. **Cost:** Assisted living facilities can be expensive, and costs can vary significantly depending on the level of care required.

3. **Loss of Home Environment:** Some individuals may feel a sense of loss or discomfort when leaving their home and moving to an assisted living facility.

The decision between home care and assisted living should be based on a thorough assessment of the individual's care needs, family resources, and the quality of available care options. In some cases, a combination of both home care and assisted living may be considered, transitioning from one to the other as the individual's needs change over time. Careful planning and regular reassessment of the chosen care arrangement are essential to ensure the individual's well-being and safety throughout their journey with Alzheimer's.
Memory Care Facilities

Chapter 9

Legal and Financial Planning

Legal and financial planning for Alzheimer's disease is crucial to ensure that individuals with the condition and their families are prepared for the complex challenges that may arise. Alzheimer's is a progressive disease that can affect decision-making capacity, making it essential to put legal and financial arrangements in place while the individual with Alzheimer's is still capable of making informed decisions. Here are key aspects of legal and financial planning for Alzheimer's:

1. **Advance Directives:** Advance directives, including a living will and durable power of attorney for healthcare, allow individuals to specify their medical preferences and designate someone to make medical decisions on their behalf if they become unable to do so. This ensures that their wishes are respected regarding life-sustaining treatments.

2. **Financial Power of Attorney:** A durable power of attorney for finances designates someone to manage financial affairs on the individual's behalf, including paying bills, managing investments, and making financial decisions. This is crucial for ensuring that financial matters are handled properly.

3. **Will and Estate Planning:** Establishing a will and estate plan helps outline how the individual's assets and property should be distributed upon their passing. It can also include provisions for guardianship of minor children and considerations for beneficiaries with special needs.

4. **Trusts:** Setting up trusts, such as revocable or irrevocable trusts, can help manage and protect assets. Trusts can be particularly useful for individuals who may require Medicaid assistance for long-term care in the future.

5. **Long-Term Care Insurance:** Investigating long-term care insurance options early can help cover the costs associated with Alzheimer's care, which can be substantial. Premiums are typically lower when purchased at a younger age.

6. **Medicaid Planning:** Medicaid is a government program that can help cover long-term care costs for individuals with limited financial resources. Proper planning and asset protection strategies may be necessary to qualify for Medicaid benefits.

7. **Beneficiary Designations:** Review and update beneficiary designations on accounts, insurance policies, and retirement plans to ensure they align with the individual's wishes.

8. **Legal Capacity Assessment:** A legal capacity assessment can help determine whether the individual with Alzheimer's has the capacity to make legal decisions. This assessment may be conducted by an attorney or a medical professional.

9. **Consultation with Professionals:** It's essential to work with legal and financial professionals who have expertise in elder law and Alzheimer's-related planning to ensure that all legal documents are valid and comply with state laws.

10. **Regular Review:** Legal and financial plans should be regularly reviewed and updated as circumstances change or as the disease progresses. This ensures that the plans remain relevant and effective.

Legal and financial planning for Alzheimer's is not only about protecting assets but also about preserving the dignity and autonomy of the individual with Alzheimer's and ensuring that their best interests are upheld. Early planning and careful consideration of all aspects of legal and financial matters are vital for individuals and their families facing Alzheimer's disease.

Advance Directives

Advance Directives are legal documents that allow individuals to express their healthcare preferences in advance, ensuring that their wishes are honored even when they may not be able to communicate or make decisions due to cognitive impairment, such as Alzheimer's disease. When it comes to Alzheimer's, these directives take on a particular significance, as the disease progresses and the individual's capacity to make informed decisions diminishes.

One of the primary components of an Advance Directive for Alzheimer's is the appointment of a healthcare proxy or durable power of attorney for healthcare. This person is designated to make medical decisions on behalf of the individual when they are no longer able to do so themselves. Selecting a trusted individual who understands the individual's values and preferences is paramount.

Additionally, individuals with Alzheimer's can outline their specific wishes regarding the type of care they desire. This may include preferences for medical interventions, end-of-life care, and the use of life-sustaining treatments. For instance, some may express a desire to receive palliative care and forgo aggressive treatments when the disease reaches an advanced stage.

In some regions, there are specialized Alzheimer's-specific Advance Directives that cater to the unique needs of individuals with this condition. These directives address issues like ongoing care, caregiver support, and residential preferences, providing comprehensive guidance for families and healthcare providers.

Advance Directives for Alzheimer's should be created early in the disease's progression when the individual is still capable of making sound decisions. It is a proactive step that can alleviate the burden of decision-making on family members and ensure that the individual's preferences are respected. Regular updates and discussions with the designated healthcare proxy are crucial to adapt the plan as the disease evolves.

In conclusion, Advance Directives play a vital role in ensuring that individuals with Alzheimer's receive care that aligns with their wishes and values, even as their cognitive abilities decline. These documents empower individuals to maintain control over their healthcare decisions and provide much-needed guidance to loved ones and healthcare professionals during a challenging journey

Managing finances

Alzheimer's disease poses significant challenges, not only to an individual's cognitive function but also to their ability to manage finances effectively. As the disease progresses, individuals with Alzheimer's may struggle with tasks like paying bills, managing bank accounts, and making sound financial decisions. Here are essential tips for managing finances when dealing with Alzheimer's:

1. Early Planning: It's crucial to start financial planning as early as possible after a diagnosis. This includes appointing a trusted family member or friend as a financial power of attorney to make financial decisions on behalf of the individual when they are no longer capable.

2. Simplify Finances: Streamline financial matters by consolidating accounts and automating bill payments. Reduce the complexity of financial tasks to minimize confusion and errors.

3. Monitor Accounts: Regularly review bank statements and financial transactions to detect any unusual activity. This can help prevent financial exploitation or fraud, which individuals with Alzheimer's are vulnerable to.

4. Create a Budget: Develop a clear budget to track income and expenses. This will help ensure that essential expenses are covered, and resources are managed efficiently.

5. Legal Documents: Work with an attorney to establish a comprehensive estate plan, including a will, living will, and trusts.

This ensures that assets are managed and distributed according to the individual's wishes.

6. Seek Professional Help: Consult with financial advisors who specialize in elder care and Alzheimer's to provide guidance on investments, long-term care insurance, and Medicaid planning.

7. Avoid Complex Investments: As the disease progresses, it's advisable to move investments into low-risk, easily understandable options. Avoid complicated investments that may be challenging to monitor.

8. Engage Family: Open communication with family members is vital. Keep them informed about financial decisions and plans, and encourage collaboration to ensure the individual's financial well-being.

9. Plan for Long-Term Care: Alzheimer's often requires long-term care, which can be costly. Explore options such as long-term care insurance or Medicaid planning to cover these expenses.

10. Stay Organized: Use tools like calendars, reminders, and financial management apps to help the individual and their caregiver stay organized and on top of financial responsibilities.

Managing finances with Alzheimer's requires proactive planning and careful consideration of the individual's changing needs. Seeking professional guidance and involving family members can help alleviate some of the stress associated with financial management, allowing the focus to remain on the well-being and quality of life of the person with Alzheimer's.

Long-Term Care Insurance

Long-term care insurance (LTCI) is a financial tool that can provide critical support for individuals with Alzheimer's disease. Alzheimer's is a progressive condition that often requires extensive care as it advances, and LTCI can help cover the substantial costs associated with long-term care services, ensuring peace of mind for both individuals and their families.

LTCI typically covers a range of care services, including in-home care, assisted living facilities, nursing homes, and memory care units, which are specifically designed for individuals with Alzheimer's and related dementias. This coverage can alleviate the financial burden on families and allow individuals to access the care they need without depleting their savings.

When considering LTCI for Alzheimer's, it's essential to plan early. Premiums are more affordable when purchased at a younger age, and individuals are more likely to be eligible for coverage before a diagnosis of Alzheimer's or other cognitive impairments. Waiting until a later stage of the disease may limit options or increase costs.

Before purchasing LTCI, it's crucial to thoroughly research policies, understand coverage limits, exclusions, waiting periods, and benefit triggers related to cognitive impairment. Consulting with a financial advisor who specializes in elder care and insurance can help individuals and their families make informed decisions about the best policy for their needs.

In summary, long-term care insurance can be a valuable investment for individuals facing Alzheimer's disease. It provides financial protection, access to quality care, and peace of mind during a challenging and uncertain time. Early planning and careful policy selection are key to maximizing the benefits of LTCI in Alzheimer's care.

Chapter 10

Coping Strategies

Coping with Alzheimer's requires patience, understanding, and a tailored approach. Here are some essential strategies:

1. Education: Learn about Alzheimer's to understand its progression and challenges.

2. Communication: Use clear, simple language, and maintain a routine to minimize confusion.

3. Support Network: Seek help from support groups and organizations specializing in Alzheimer's care.

4. Self-Care: Caregivers should prioritize their well-being, seeking respite and assistance when needed.

5. Safety: Make necessary home modifications and ensure a safe environment.

6. Memory Aids: Use memory aids like calendars and reminders.

7. Flexibility: Adapt to changing needs and be prepared for mood swings or behavioral changes.

8. Legal Planning: Establish legal documents like Advance Directives and power of attorney.

9. Enjoyment: Engage in activities the individual enjoys, promoting a higher quality of life.

10. Patience: Be patient, empathetic, and focus on preserving dignity throughout the journey.

Emotional Support

Emotional support is a cornerstone of care for individuals living with Alzheimer's disease. The emotional challenges that accompany cognitive decline can be just as significant as the physical ones. Here are key elements of emotional support for Alzheimer's:

1. **Empathy and Understanding:** Acknowledge the person's feelings and experiences, even if they cannot express them clearly. Show empathy and patience.

2. **Open Communication:** Encourage communication, even if it's non-verbal. Maintain eye contact, listen actively, and respond with kindness.

3. **Validation:** Validate the individual's emotions and experiences, even if they don't align with reality. It helps reduce distress and confusion.

4. **Routine and Familiarity:** Maintain a consistent routine and surround the person with familiar objects and people. Predictability can reduce anxiety.

5. **Social Engagement:** Encourage social interaction with friends and family to combat feelings of isolation and depression.

6. **Sensory Stimulation:** Engage the senses through music, touch, or aromatherapy, which can evoke positive emotions and memories.

7. **Respect and Dignity:** Treat the person with Alzheimer's with respect and uphold their dignity at all times, even in challenging situations.

8. **Caregiver Support:** Caregivers also need emotional support. Seek help from support groups or professionals to manage stress and burnout.

9. **Creative Outlets:** Explore creative activities like art, storytelling, or gardening, which can provide emotional expression and fulfillment.

10. **Future Planning:** Involve the person in discussions about their future care to give them a sense of control and involvement.

Emotional support plays a pivotal role in enhancing the quality of life for both individuals with Alzheimer's and their caregivers. By fostering an environment of empathy, understanding, and patience, it's possible to create a more compassionate and nurturing caregiving experience.

Maintaining Quality of Life

A diagnosis of Alzheimer's disease can be daunting, but with a holistic approach, individuals and their caregivers can strive to maintain a good quality of life throughout the journey. Here are key strategies:

1. **Early Diagnosis and Planning:** Early diagnosis allows for better planning. Create Advance Directives and establish a support network.

2. **Physical Health:** Encourage a healthy lifestyle with balanced nutrition and regular exercise to support overall well-being.

3. **Mental Stimulation:** Engage the mind with puzzles, memory games, and social interactions to stimulate cognitive function.

4. **Routine and Familiarity:** Maintain a consistent daily routine and surround the individual with familiar objects and people to reduce anxiety.

5. **Emotional Support:** Provide emotional support through open communication, empathy, and validation of feelings.

6. **Safety Measures:** Ensure a safe home environment with necessary modifications to prevent accidents.

7. **Social Engagement:** Foster social connections through visits with friends, family, or participation in support groups.

8. **Creative Expression:** Encourage creative outlets like art, music, or storytelling, which can provide emotional expression and joy.

9. **Respect and Dignity:** Uphold the person's dignity and treat them with respect in all interactions.

10. **Self-Care for Caregivers:** Caregivers should prioritize their own well-being, seeking respite and support when needed to prevent burnout.

11. **Medication and Therapies:** Consult with healthcare professionals for medication and therapies that can help manage symptoms.

12. **End-of-Life Planning:** Discuss end-of-life preferences and decisions while the individual can still participate.

While Alzheimer's presents unique challenges, a comprehensive approach that addresses physical, mental, emotional, and social aspects can help individuals and their caregivers navigate the journey with dignity and enhance their overall quality of life. It's essential to adapt strategies as the disease progresses to meet changing needs and promote well-being.

Building a Support Network

Caring for someone with Alzheimer's disease is a challenging and often long-term endeavor that requires a strong support network. Building and maintaining such a network is crucial for the well-being of both the individual with Alzheimer's and their caregivers. Here's how to create a supportive network for Alzheimer's care:

1. **Family and Friends:** Start by reaching out to close family members and friends who can provide emotional support, respite care, and assistance with daily tasks. They can form the core of your caregiving team.

2. **Support Groups:** Join local or online Alzheimer's support groups where you can connect with others facing similar challenges. These groups offer valuable advice, share experiences, and provide a sense of community.

3. **Healthcare Professionals:** Build strong relationships with healthcare providers, including doctors, nurses, and specialists. They can offer guidance on treatment options, symptom management, and medical care.

4. **Home Care Services:** Consider hiring professional caregivers or home healthcare services to provide assistance with daily activities, allowing you to take breaks and maintain your own well-being.

5. **Community Resources:** Explore community resources such as senior centers, adult day programs, and meal delivery services. These can offer respite for caregivers and social engagement for the individual with Alzheimer's.

6. **Legal and Financial Advisors:** Consult with legal and financial professionals to ensure you have the necessary documents in place, such as power of attorney and Advance Directives. They can also provide advice on managing finances and navigating government assistance programs.

7. **Alzheimer's Associations:** Organizations like the Alzheimer's Association offer a wealth of information, resources, and

educational programs. They can connect you with local services and events.

8. **Faith-Based Communities:** For those who are religious, faith-based communities can provide emotional support and assistance, including pastoral care.

9. **Respite Care:** Arrange for regular respite care, either through family members, friends, or professional caregivers, to give yourself much-needed breaks to recharge.

10. **Technology:** Utilize technology to stay connected and informed. There are apps and devices designed to assist with medication management, tracking daily routines, and ensuring safety.

11. **Stay Informed:** Continuously educate yourself about Alzheimer's disease, its progression, and caregiving strategies. Knowledge empowers you to make informed decisions.

12. **Open Communication:** Maintain open and honest communication within your network. Share updates, concerns, and needs to ensure everyone is on the same page.

Creating and nurturing a supportive network for Alzheimer's care is an ongoing process. Regularly assess your needs, adjust your network, and don't hesitate to ask for help. A strong support system can help alleviate the challenges of Alzheimer's caregiving, providing emotional, physical, and practical assistance along the journey.

Chapter 11

Research and Hope

Alzheimer's disease, a devastating neurodegenerative condition, has long been a focus of intense research efforts, offering a glimmer of hope for millions affected worldwide. Here are key reasons for optimism in Alzheimer's research:

1. **Increased Funding:** Governments, nonprofits, and private organizations have substantially increased funding for Alzheimer's research, driving progress in understanding the disease's mechanisms.

2. **Early Detection:** Advances in neuroimaging and biomarker development are enabling earlier and more accurate diagnosis, allowing for timely intervention and treatment.

3. **Clinical Trials:** A growing number of clinical trials are testing potential therapies and interventions to slow, halt, or even reverse Alzheimer's progression, offering promising avenues for treatment.

4. **Diverse Approaches:** Researchers are exploring various approaches, from drugs targeting amyloid plaques and tau protein tangles to lifestyle interventions, immunotherapies, and precision medicine.

5. **Prevention Focus:** There's increasing emphasis on prevention strategies, such as lifestyle modifications (diet, exercise, cognitive engagement), to reduce Alzheimer's risk.

6. **Collaboration:** Global collaboration among researchers, institutions, and pharmaceutical companies is accelerating the pace of discovery and innovation.

7. **Genetic Insights:** Genetic research has revealed key risk factors, aiding in the development of personalized treatment approaches for those at higher genetic risk.

8. **Patient Advocacy:** Advocacy groups and Alzheimer's associations are championing the cause, raising awareness, and driving policy changes to support research and care.

9. **Technological Advances:** Cutting-edge technologies like artificial intelligence and big data analysis are aiding in the identification of potential drug targets and early disease markers.

10. **Care Improvements:** Research isn't just focused on a cure; it's also improving the quality of care and support services available to individuals and families affected by Alzheimer's.

While a definitive cure for Alzheimer's remains elusive, the collective efforts of the global scientific community offer hope that more effective treatments, prevention strategies, and improved care will emerge. Alzheimer's research continues to advance, bringing us closer to a future where this devastating disease can be more effectively managed and, ultimately, conquered. Hope remains a driving force in the quest to understand and combat Alzheimer's.

Current Research and Breakthroughs

Current Research and Breakthroughs in Alzheimer's Disease

Alzheimer's disease research has witnessed significant advancements in recent years, offering hope for better understanding, early detection, and potential treatments. Some notable breakthroughs and ongoing research areas include:

1. **Amyloid-Targeting Drugs:** Several promising drugs are in development to target amyloid plaques, a hallmark of Alzheimer's. Aducanumab, approved by the FDA in 2021, is one such breakthrough, although its effectiveness remains a subject of debate.

2. **Tau Protein Therapies:** Researchers are exploring drugs that target tau protein tangles, another key pathological feature of Alzheimer's. These therapies aim to slow or halt disease progression.

3. **Blood Biomarkers:** Advances in identifying blood-based biomarkers for Alzheimer's are making early detection more feasible, potentially allowing for interventions before symptoms become severe.

4. **Immunotherapies:** Innovative immunotherapies are being developed to boost the immune system's ability to clear amyloid and tau proteins from the brain.

5. **Precision Medicine:** Tailoring treatments to individuals based on their genetic, biological, and lifestyle factors is an emerging trend in Alzheimer's research, with the goal of achieving more personalized and effective therapies.

6. **Lifestyle Interventions:** Studies continue to emphasize the importance of lifestyle factors, such as diet, exercise, and cognitive engagement, in reducing Alzheimer's risk and managing symptoms.

7. **Neuroinflammation:** Researchers are exploring the role of neuroinflammation in Alzheimer's and potential anti-inflammatory treatments.

8. **Technology and Artificial Intelligence:** Advanced imaging techniques, data analysis, and artificial intelligence are aiding in early diagnosis, tracking disease progression, and identifying new therapeutic targets.

9. **Gene Editing:** Emerging gene-editing technologies like CRISPR hold potential for modifying genes associated with Alzheimer's risk.

10. **Global Collaborations:** International research collaborations and data-sharing initiatives are accelerating progress by pooling resources and expertise.

While a definitive cure remains elusive, these breakthroughs and ongoing research efforts offer optimism in the fight against Alzheimer's. They bring us closer to a future where early detection, targeted therapies, and effective interventions can significantly improve the lives of those affected by this devastating disease.

Clinical Trials

Clinical trials are pivotal in the quest to unravel the complexities of Alzheimer's disease and develop effective treatments. These research studies involve testing potential therapies, interventions, and diagnostic tools to better understand the disease and improve patient outcomes. Here are key aspects of clinical trials in Alzheimer's:

1. **Diverse Targets:** Clinical trials explore a wide range of approaches, from drugs targeting amyloid plaques

Promising Treatments

As the scientific community intensifies its efforts to combat Alzheimer's disease, several promising treatments have emerged on the horizon, providing hope for individuals and families affected by this devastating condition. Here are some notable approaches showing potential:

1. **Anti-Amyloid Therapies:** Alzheimer's is characterized by the accumulation of amyloid plaques in the brain. Several drugs are in development that aim to either clear existing plaques or prevent

their formation. Aducanumab, while met with controversy, is a pioneering example.

2. **Tau Protein Targeting:** Tau protein tangles are another hallmark of Alzheimer's. Therapies focused on reducing or clearing tau pathology are showing promise in preclinical and early clinical studies.

3. **Anti-Inflammatory Agents:** Chronic inflammation in the brain is believed to play a role in Alzheimer's progression. Drugs targeting neuroinflammation are being investigated for their potential to slow the disease.

4. **Immunotherapies:** Immunotherapies aim to harness the immune system to target and remove abnormal proteins associated with Alzheimer's, offering a novel approach to treatment.

5. **Lifestyle Interventions:** Lifestyle modifications, including diet, exercise, and cognitive engagement, have demonstrated potential in reducing Alzheimer's risk and managing symptoms, emphasizing the importance of holistic approaches.

6. **Precision Medicine:** Tailoring treatments based on individual genetics and biological factors is an emerging strategy to achieve more personalized and effective therapies.

7. **Gene Editing:** Cutting-edge gene-editing techniques like CRISPR hold promise for modifying genes associated with Alzheimer's risk, potentially preventing or mitigating the disease.

8. **Combination Therapies:** Researchers are exploring the synergistic effects of combining different treatment approaches to enhance their effectiveness.

While none of these treatments has yet led to a definitive cure, the progress in Alzheimer's research offers hope that a breakthrough may be on the horizon. Clinical trials continue to be a critical avenue for testing these treatments and pushing the boundaries of our understanding of Alzheimer's disease. As research advances, the goal remains to provide better care, slow progression, and ultimately find a cure for this challenging condition.

Future Directions

The future of Alzheimer's disease research and care holds great promise, driven by ongoing scientific advancements and a growing understanding of this complex condition. Here are key directions that will shape the future of Alzheimer's:

1. **Early Detection and Diagnosis:** Innovations in biomarker research and neuroimaging techniques will lead to earlier and more accurate detection of Alzheimer's, allowing for timely intervention and personalized treatment plans.

2. **Precision Medicine:** Tailoring treatments based on individual genetics and biological factors will become more common, allowing for targeted therapies that match each patient's unique needs and characteristics.

3. **Disease-Modifying Therapies:** Advances in drug development will continue to target the underlying mechanisms of Alzheimer's, with a focus on halting or slowing disease progression rather than just alleviating symptoms.

4. **Comprehensive Care Models:** Holistic approaches that incorporate not only medical treatments but also lifestyle modifications, cognitive interventions, and emotional support will become standard in Alzheimer's care.

5. **Technological Solutions:** Smart devices, telehealth, and artificial intelligence will play a more significant role in managing and monitoring Alzheimer's patients, enhancing caregiving and improving patient outcomes.

6. **Global Collaboration:** Collaborative efforts between researchers, institutions, and governments worldwide will accelerate progress, allowing for more effective data sharing and resource allocation.

7. **Patient Advocacy:** Advocacy groups and individuals affected by Alzheimer's will continue to push for increased research funding, policy changes, and improved access to care and support services.

8. **Prevention Focus:** Public health initiatives will emphasize lifestyle modifications to reduce Alzheimer's risk, targeting factors such as diet, exercise, and mental stimulation.

9. **Ethical Considerations:** As treatments become more personalized, ethical questions surrounding genetic testing, data privacy, and informed consent will require careful consideration and regulation.

10. **Cultivating Hope:** The search for a cure remains steadfast, with optimism fueled by a deeper understanding of the disease and the determination to improve the lives of those impacted by Alzheimer's.

In the coming years, these future directions will continue to shape the landscape of Alzheimer's research and care, offering hope for more effective treatments, better quality of life for individuals with Alzheimer's, and ultimately, the pursuit of a cure for this challenging condition.

Chapter 12

Caregiving Perspective

Caring for someone with Alzheimer's disease is a deeply challenging journey, one that requires immense patience, empathy, and resilience. From the caregiver's perspective, it is a rollercoaster of emotions, from moments of heartwarming connection to heart-wrenching frustration.

One of the key aspects of caregiving for Alzheimer's patients is the gradual loss of memory and cognitive function. Caregivers often witness their loved ones struggle with basic tasks they once mastered, like dressing or eating. This can be emotionally taxing as they grapple with the cruel progression of the disease, knowing that there is no cure.

Moreover, caregivers must adapt to ever-changing behaviors and mood swings. Alzheimer's can cause agitation, confusion, and even aggression in patients. Caregivers must learn to respond with compassion, seeking to understand the underlying fears or discomfort that trigger these outbursts.

On the flip side, there are moments of profound connection. A smile, a flicker of recognition, or a shared memory can be incredibly rewarding for caregivers. These moments remind them of the person they are caring for, beyond the disease.

Ultimately, the caregiving perspective on Alzheimer's is a complex mix of sorrow and love, exhaustion and devotion. It requires a network of support, self-care, and an unwavering commitment to preserving dignity and comfort for those living with this relentless condition.

Personal Stories

Personal stories of Alzheimer's disease offer profound insights into the impact of this condition on individuals and their families. These narratives shed light on the emotional and practical challenges faced by those affected.

In these stories, individuals diagnosed with Alzheimer's often describe the gradual erosion of their memories and identity. They share the frustration of forgetting names, places, and even the faces of loved ones. These accounts underscore the importance of early diagnosis and the pursuit of meaningful experiences while they can still be enjoyed.

Family members who care for loved ones with Alzheimer's share their journeys too. They talk about the heartache of witnessing cognitive decline and the delicate balance of providing support while respecting their autonomy. These stories emphasize the need for patience, empathy, and adaptability in caregiving.

Importantly, personal stories also highlight the resilience and strength found in unexpected places. Many individuals with Alzheimer's continue to find joy in music, art, and simple daily routines. Caregivers often discover new depths of compassion and love amidst the challenges.

These narratives serve as a reminder of the urgent need for more research, funding, and support for Alzheimer's patients and their families. They inspire hope that, even in the face of a devastating disease, moments of connection, understanding, and love can endure.

Coping as a Caregiver

Coping as a caregiver for someone with Alzheimer's is a demanding and emotionally charged journey. It requires resilience, patience, and self-care to navigate the unique challenges this role presents.

First and foremost, caregivers must educate themselves about Alzheimer's disease. Understanding its progression, symptoms, and available resources is crucial for providing effective care. Support groups, online communities, and caregiver training programs can be invaluable sources of information and emotional support.

Emotional resilience is paramount. Alzheimer's can be emotionally taxing as caregivers witness their loved ones' decline. It's essential to acknowledge the sadness, frustration, and even anger that may arise and seek outlets for these emotions, whether through therapy, journaling, or confiding in trusted friends and family.

Creating a structured routine can help both the caregiver and the individual with Alzheimer's. Predictable daily schedules provide a sense of security and reduce confusion for the patient. Additionally, caregivers must practice patience and flexibility as they adapt to changing behaviors and needs.

Respite care is vital for caregivers' well-being. Taking breaks, even if short, allows caregivers to recharge and prevent burnout. Friends and family should be encouraged to step in and offer support.

Above all, self-compassion is crucial. Caregivers must acknowledge their limitations and accept that they cannot control the progression of the disease. Seeking professional help when needed and remembering that they are doing their best under challenging circumstances can help caregivers cope with the profound challenges of caring for someone with Alzheimer's.

Finding Joy in the Journey

Finding joy in the journey of Alzheimer's, while undoubtedly challenging, is a testament to the strength of the human spirit and the power of love and connection. Amidst the turmoil of this progressive disease, there are moments of beauty and happiness waiting to be discovered.

One source of joy is the ability to create new, meaningful memories. Alzheimer's may erase old recollections, but it doesn't extinguish the capacity for new experiences. Caregivers can find delight in simple pleasures, like a shared laugh, a comforting touch, or a favorite song that sparks recognition.

Music and art often become powerful tools for unlocking moments of joy. Familiar melodies can rekindle forgotten memories, and creative activities can provide a sense of accomplishment and self-expression for individuals with Alzheimer's.

Another source of joy lies in the resilience and adaptability of those affected by Alzheimer's. Their ability to find contentment in the present moment, free from the burdens of the past or anxieties about the future, can be inspiring. Caregivers witness the beauty of unconditional love, as they provide support and care despite the challenges.

Ultimately, finding joy in the Alzheimer's journey is about embracing the moments of connection, tenderness, and shared humanity. It's about celebrating the person beyond the disease, cherishing the glimpses of recognition, and holding onto the love that endures despite memory's fading grasp. In these moments, the journey becomes not just a struggle but a testament to the enduring power of love and the resilience of the human spirit.

Chapter 13

Alzheimer's Advocacy and Awareness

Alzheimer's advocacy and awareness efforts are critical in addressing the profound impact of this disease on individuals, families, and society as a whole. By raising awareness and advocating for change, we can work towards a world where Alzheimer's is better understood, diagnosed earlier, and ultimately, cured.

Advocacy for Alzheimer's focuses on several key areas:

1. Research Funding: Advocacy efforts aim to secure increased funding for Alzheimer's research. Continued investment is essential to understand the disease's causes, develop effective treatments, and ultimately find a cure.

2. Early Detection and Diagnosis: Raising awareness about the importance of early detection and diagnosis can lead to more individuals seeking help in the early stages of the disease, enabling better management and planning.

3. Support for Caregivers: Alzheimer's advocacy emphasizes the need for support services and resources for caregivers who play a crucial role in the lives of those affected. This includes access to respite care, educational programs, and emotional support.

4. Reducing Stigma: Advocacy campaigns work to reduce the stigma associated with Alzheimer's, promoting understanding and empathy for individuals living with the disease and their caregivers.

5. Public Policy: Advocates engage with policymakers to influence legislation that addresses the needs of Alzheimer's patients and their families, including improved access to healthcare services and long-term care options.

By raising awareness and advocating for these issues, we can create a more compassionate and informed society that is better equipped to address the challenges of Alzheimer's disease and ultimately improve the lives of those affected by it.

Joining the Fight

Joining the fight against Alzheimer's is a call to action that can make a profound difference in the lives of millions affected by this devastating disease. It's a commitment to support research, raise awareness, and provide care for those living with Alzheimer's and their caregivers.

1. **Supporting Research**: One of the most impactful ways to join the fight is by contributing to Alzheimer's research. Donations to research organizations fund studies seeking to understand the disease's causes and develop effective treatments or, ideally, a cure. Advocating for increased research funding can also make a significant impact.

2. **Raising Awareness**: Spreading awareness about Alzheimer's is crucial to reduce stigma and encourage early diagnosis. Engage in conversations, share educational materials, and participate in Alzheimer's awareness events to help others understand the challenges faced by individuals and families.

3. **Volunteering**: Many organizations focused on Alzheimer's rely on volunteers to provide support and resources to affected individuals and caregivers. Volunteering your time and skills can have a direct, positive impact on those dealing with the disease.

4. **Advocacy**: Joining advocacy groups and initiatives can influence policy changes that benefit Alzheimer's patients and caregivers. By advocating for increased research funding, better access to care, and improved support services, you can help shape a more compassionate and effective response to the disease.

5. **Supporting Caregivers**: Offer your assistance and empathy to caregivers, as they often face physical and emotional strain. Providing respite care or simply being there to listen and support can make a significant difference in their lives.

By joining the fight against Alzheimer's, you become part of a global community dedicated to improving the quality of life for those affected and working towards a future where Alzheimer's is no longer a devastating diagnosis. Your involvement, whether through donations, volunteering, advocacy, or support, contributes to this important cause.

Raising Awareness

Raising awareness about Alzheimer's disease is crucial in our society. Alzheimer's is a progressive and debilitating brain disorder that affects millions of individuals worldwide, along with their families and caregivers. To combat the challenges posed by this condition, it is imperative to promote understanding, empathy, and early detection.

Firstly, awareness campaigns can educate the public about the early signs of Alzheimer's, such as memory loss, confusion, and changes in behavior. Recognizing these symptoms is vital for early intervention, potentially slowing the disease's progression.

Secondly, raising awareness reduces stigma. Many individuals with Alzheimer's face discrimination and isolation due to misconceptions about the disease. By dispelling these myths, society can become more inclusive and supportive of those affected.

Thirdly, increased awareness can drive funding and research efforts. With more people informed about the impact of Alzheimer's, governments, organizations, and individuals are more likely to invest in research for better treatments and, ultimately, a cure.

In conclusion, raising awareness about Alzheimer's is a crucial step in improving the lives of those affected by this devastating disease. By fostering understanding, empathy, and financial support, we can work together to provide a brighter future for individuals and families living with Alzheimer's.

The Road Ahead

The road ahead in the battle against Alzheimer's disease is both challenging and hopeful. While there are still many mysteries surrounding this devastating condition, there are several promising avenues of progress that offer hope for the future.

Firstly, research into Alzheimer's is advancing rapidly. Scientists are gaining a deeper understanding of the disease's mechanisms, genetic factors, and risk factors. This knowledge is crucial in developing effective treatments and, ultimately, a cure.

Secondly, early detection and intervention are becoming more feasible. Advances in brain imaging and biomarker research are enabling doctors to diagnose Alzheimer's at earlier stages, providing a window of opportunity for intervention and potential lifestyle changes that may slow the disease's progression.

Thirdly, there is a growing emphasis on providing support for caregivers. Caring for a loved one with Alzheimer's can be physically and emotionally taxing. Initiatives are emerging to provide caregivers with resources, respite, and education to better manage the challenges they face.

However, significant hurdles remain. Alzheimer's research requires substantial funding, and the caregiving burden will continue to grow as the aging population increases. Societal awareness and advocacy will be crucial in pushing for more resources and a comprehensive approach to addressing Alzheimer's.

In conclusion, while the road ahead in the fight against Alzheimer's disease is challenging, there is reason for optimism. With continued research, early detection, caregiver support, and public awareness, we can work toward a future where Alzheimer's is better understood and, ultimately, conquered.

www.ingramcontent.com/pod-product-compliance
Lightning Source LLC
Chambersburg PA
CBHW071608270726
48661CB00019B/1648